THE
WHOLE GRAIN
PROMISE

More Than 100 Delicious Recipes
to Jumpstart a Healthier Diet

ROBIN ASBELL

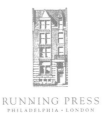

RUNNING PRESS
PHILADELPHIA · LONDON

Published by Running Press,
A Member of the Perseus Books Group

Books published by Running Press are available at special discounts for bulk purchases in the
United States by corporations, institutions, and other organizations. For more information, please
contact the Special Markets Department at the Perseus Books Group, 2300 Chestnut Street, Suite 200,
Philadelphia, PA 19103, or call (800) 810-4145, ext. 5000, or e-mail special.markets@perseusbooks.com.

ISBN 978-0-7624-5662-8
Library of Congress Control Number: 2015934362
E-book ISBN 978-0-7624-5810-3

9 8 7 6 5 4 3 2 1
Digit on the right indicates the number of this printing

Designed by Amanda Richmond
Edited by Zachary Leibman
Food Styling by Carrie Purcell
Prop Styling by Mariellen Melker
Typography: Burford, Sentinel, and Whitney

Running Press Book Publishers
2300 Chestnut Street
Philadelphia, PA 19103–4371

Visit us on the web!
www.offthemenublog.com

⚓

CONTENTS

INTRODUCTION ... **7**

HEALTH BENEFITS ... **11**

THE PSYCHOLOGY OF "HEALTHY FOOD" ... **12**

GETTING STARTED ... **14**

STRATEGIES FOR MAKING IT EASY (AND SAVING MONEY) ... **17**

GLOSSARY OF GRAINS AND FLOURS ... **23**

BREAKFAST...**28**

Soaks, Overnights, and Boil-and-Leave-in-the-Pan Cereals ... 29

Overnight Oat Soak with Pomegranate, Berries, and Nuts ... 29

Boil-and-Leave Steel-Cut Oats ... 30

Quick Stovetop Granola ... 31

Super-Chunky Sweet Cherry-Almond Granola ... 32

Daily Walnut-Raisin Olive Oil Granola ... 33

Date and Grain Energy Bars ... 34

Three Super Smoothies: Blueberry Green Smoothie with Leftover Grain, Strawberry-Banana Quinoa Smoothie, and Granola Island Smoothie ... 35

Lemon-Strawberry Quinoa Breakfast Salad ... 37

Farro with Clementines and Yogurt Dressing ... 38

Leftover-Grain Omelets and Scrambles ... 40

Grilled Steel-Cut Oat Slabs with Sautéed Apples ... 41

Asian Breakfast Bowls: Japanese Breakfast Bowl and Egg Curry Breakfast Bowl ... 43

Savory Porridge ... 45

Cinnamon Toast and Fruit "Caprese" ... 46

Pumpkin Pie Baked Steel-Cut Oats ... 47

Peachy Yogurt Coffee Cake ... 48

Cinnamon–Apple Butter Bars ... 50

Fruity Carrot Muffins ... 51

Yogurt–Cottage Cheese Muffins with Tarragon ... 52

Cherry and Pine Nut Breakfast Focaccia ... 53

Breakfast Pizza with Strawberry Sauce, Ricotta, and Sweet Walnut "Meatballs" ... 54

Biscuit-Topped Breakfast Pie ... 55

Puffy Baked Apple Pancake ... 56

Big Cinnamon-Oat Pancakes with Berries ... 57

Overnight Whole Wheat Waffles with Maple-Pear Sauce ... 59

BREADS...**60**

Make Your Own Baking Mix ... 61

Baking-Mix Biscuits ... 62

Baking-Mix Pancakes ... 62

Baking-Mix Scones ... 63

No-Knead "Stealth" Bread ... 64

Overnight "Stealth" Pizza Dough . . . 67

Soft Buttermilk Buns . . . 68

Savory Granola Croutons for Salad or Soup . . . 69

Basic Croutons with Variations . . . 70

Savory Spinach Quick Bread . . . 71

Cheddar-Chive Cornbread . . . 73

Cherry-Almond Quick Bread . . . 74

Parsley-Parmesan Popovers . . . 77

SALADS . . . 78

Kale and Tomato Caesar Salad . . . 79

Italian Bread Salad . . . 80

Buddha Bowls for Two . . . 81

Mixed Rice Cobb with Avocados, Blue
Cheese, and Creamy Tomato Dressing . . . 82

Roasted Cauliflower, Carrots, and Parmesan
Croutons over Spinach . . . 83

Spinach Quattro Salad—Four Salads
on One Plate . . . 84

Wheat Berry and Shredded Cabbage Salad
with Buttermilk Dressing . . . 85

Middle Eastern Freekeh Salad with
Sesame-Yogurt Dressing . . . 86

Italian Farro and White Bean Salad
with Asparagus . . . 89

Sushi Broccoli and Brown Rice Salad . . . 90

Soba or Whole Wheat Spaghetti with
Sesame Dressing and Sugar Snap Peas . . . 91

Lime Quinoa Salad with Avocado
and Mango . . . 92

Wild Rice, Pear, and Roasted Sweet
Potato Salad with Walnuts . . . 95

SOUPS . . . 96

Quick Veggie Chili with Mushrooms
and Bulgur . . . 97

Creamy Curried Carrot-Millet
Soup with Mint . . . 98

Creamy Spinach Soup . . . 100

Fast Chicken Soup with Quinoa . . . 101

Spring Veggie Stew with Bulgur . . . 103

Beet and Buckwheat Borscht with
Parsley-Yogurt Garnish . . . 104

Summer Tomato-Zucchini Soup with
Wheat Berries . . . 106

Millet-Corn Chowder with Chipotle . . . 107

Mexican Tortilla Soup with Shrimp . . . 108

Spicy Cabbage Soup with Leftover-Grain
Dumplings . . . 109

SIDES . . . 110

Easy Bulgur Herb Pilaf . . . 111

Quick Lemony Couscous with Spinach . . . 112

Herbed Bread Stuffing . . . 113

Easy Basil Baked Polenta Rounds . . . 114

Whole Wheat Angel Hair with
Arugula-Ricotta Pesto . . . 115

Whole Wheat Penne in Roasted-Pepper
Romesco Sauce . . . 116

Whole Wheat Spaghetti with Garlicky
Breadcrumbs, Kale, and Parmesan . . . 117

Whole Grain Mac and Cheese with Peas . . . 119

Savory Spinach and Cheese
Bread Pudding . . . 120

Whole Grain Sour Cream and Dill Noodles . . . 121

Savory Kasha with Parsnips . . . 122

Indian Yellow Mixed-Grain Biryani . . . 125

Veggie and Brown Rice Medley . . . 126

Any-Grain Fried "Rice" with Veggies
and Egg . . . 127

Barley and Sweet Potato Timbales . . . 128

Quinoa and Sun-Dried Tomato Timbales . . . 130

Potato-Grain Croquettes with Warm
Honey-Mustard Sauce . . . 131

MAIN COURSES...132

Easy Black Bean Burgers with Oats and Avocado Salsa...133

Pecan and Barley Burgers with Peach Ketchup...135

Quinoa-Feta Phyllo Triangles...136

Lime Fish Cakes with Brown Rice and Dipping Sauce...137

Red Quinoa–Crusted Baked Fish with Cucumber-Lime Salsa...138

Baked Sole Filled with Lemony Dill Pilaf...140

Grain and Nut Balls with Marinara and Whole Wheat Penne...141

Pesto Turkey Loaf with Oats...142

Easy Black Bean Quesadillas with Raspberry-Kiwi Salsa...143

Savory Streusel Squash Pie with Oat Crust...145

Chipotle and Avocado Grain and Turkey Wraps...146

Grain-Crust Spinach Cauliflower Quiche...147

Smoky Bacon and Grain Frittata...148

Crunchy-Crumb Chicken Fingers with Honey Mustard...150

Brown Rice California Rolls with Salmon...151

Cornbread-Topped Chili Casserole...152

QUICK SNACKS...157

Super Popcorns: Peanut Butter Corn, Cinnamon Corn, and Parmesan Corn...155

Graham Sams: Graham Crackers with Chocolate Hazelnut, Almond-Apricot Spread, Maple Ricotta with Mini Chocolate Chips, and Apples and Cheddar...158

Graham Cracker and Pudding "Pie"...159

Whole Grain Cracker, Chex, and Nut Mixes: Creamy Buttermilk and Thai Chili Lime...160

Cinnamon Toasts with Yogurt Dip...161

Baked Corn Chips with Easy Edamame Hummus...162

Yogurt-Granola Parfait with Seasonal Fruit...163

Whole Wheat Pita Pizzas...164

Leftover-Grain Scallion Cakes with Curry Ketchup...167

Rice Cake Tuna Melts...168

Savory Oatmeal Cookies with Cheddar...169

DESSERTS...170

Granola Bark...171

Granola Brittle Chunks...172

"Raw" Cookie Dough Bites...173

Quick Stovetop Nectarine-Berry Crumble...174

Oatmeal and Mixed-Fruit Jumbo Cookies...175

Chewy Chocolate Cookies...176

Light Buckwheat Brownies...178

Apple Butter–Swirl Cupcakes with Cider Glaze...179

Peanut Butter Cake with Chocolate Frosting...180

Cherry-Almond Grain Pudding...181

Cranberry Cornmeal Upside-Down Cake...183

Orange-Raspberry Bundt...184

Cherry Cheesecake Bars with Extra Graham Crunch...187

Fudgy Brownie Cupcakes...188

ACKNOWLEDGMENTS...189

INDEX...190

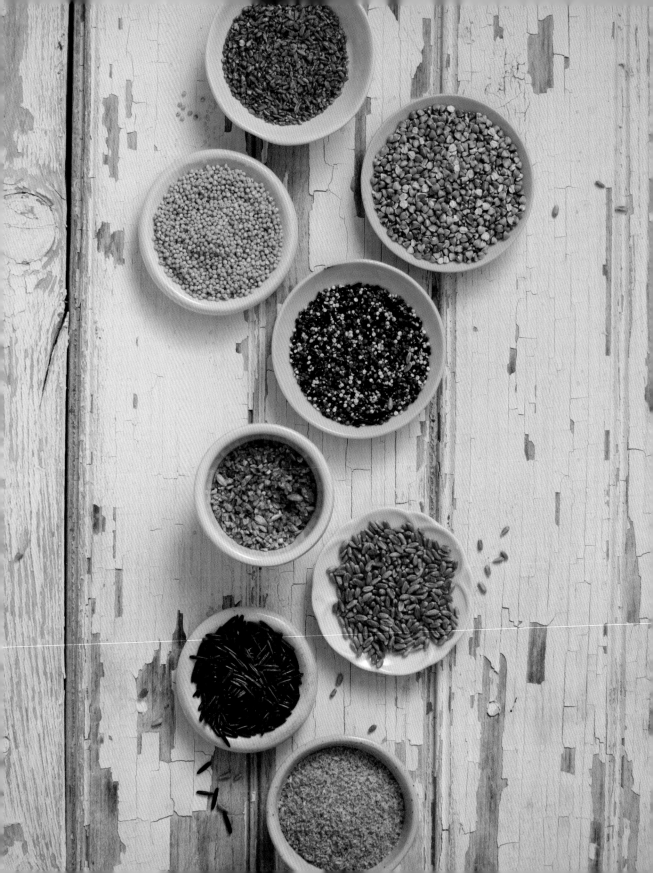

INTRODUCTION

I F WHOLE GRAINS ARE NEW TO YOU, WELCOME. YOU ARE EMBARKING ON AN ADVENTURE, filled with new flavors, textures, and renewed energy. If whole grains are familiar and you seek a spark of inspiration, you are in the right place.

This book is going to make whole grains so easy and appealing that you won't be able to imagine life without them. With grains, crave-worthy, intensely gratifying food that nourishes you deeply is an everyday miracle.

You see, the last several years have seen a revolution in the world of whole grains. Back in 2006, the USDA raised their recommendation for the consumption of whole grains from one serving a day to three, and ever since, the whole grain business has been booming. In the year 2010 alone, twenty times more whole grain products were launched worldwide than in 2000.

It's pretty amazing that a food that has formed the backbone of human diets in many regions of the world for 10,000 years could suddenly take a star turn. But everything old is new again, and fresh, exciting things are happening for whole grain foods.

The weight of all the evidence has reached critical mass, and we know that shifting more of our grain consumption to whole grains is a powerful way to improve health. Because of this exciting opportunity to improve the quality of human life with one simple change, inspired farmers, food manufacturers, artisanal bakers, chefs, and food writers like me have been working on bringing you the most appealing, interesting whole grain foods imaginable. Along the way, we've learned more about the chemistry of how food works and the techniques that create the most flavorful, exciting whole grain products and recipes.

Both artisan and industrial bakers have learned a great deal about what goes into a great loaf of whole wheat bread, whether you want a fluffy, light one or a hefty, crusty one. Pasta makers have figured out how to mix and shape whole wheat pasta with a bite and texture just like the old white flour kind. High-quality, diverse whole grain flours like white whole wheat and ancient and heritage wheats, as well as gluten-free options, are easier to find than ever. What started out as just plugging whole grains into the same dishes that we used to make with white flour evolved into a celebration of flavor as innovators learned what whole grains really taste like and how to complement those unique flavors. The creative people who bring you new foods discovered some ancient grains that deserve to be known and loved again, and they have created updated ways to prepare them.

Sure, whole grains are good for us. Don't hold that against them. We are celebrating them for their glorious, sensual wonders. Come join the party.

Believe me, if the interest in whole grains were just about health, they would have remained in their niche as "health food" and never have gone mainstream. This new excitement has grown because grains are uniquely delicious and deserve to be stars of the plate. From the crunchy wheat berry, with its sweet, tender center, to the creamy teff grain, with its subtle notes of cocoa, each grain has unique and seductive qualities. Who needs white rice when you have nutty, fragrant brown rice, sweet and earthy black rice, or Wehani red rice, with its hint of chestnuts and spice? If you want a beautifully composed plate or a gorgeous bed for a simple piece of fish or meat, nothing beats whole grains. Whether cooked plain, made into a simple pilaf, or molded into a timbale, grains make your meals pop on the plate.

The amazing, exciting, and delicious world of whole grain foods is waiting for you. These ancient, nourishing foods are still the basis of an energizing and satisfying diet, just as they have been for thousands of years. The only thing that has changed is that we now have access to far more options than our forebears did, both good and bad.

That's right, the people of northern China who grew millet 10,000 years ago would have been thrilled to try black rice or teff or a box of good whole wheat pasta. The ancient Roman gladiators, who fought epic battles fueled by barley gruel, would likely have marched a hundred miles for the loaf of whole wheat bread you can pick up at the corner store.

Much has happened in the world of whole grains since those earliest adopters first built their foodways around grain. We industrialized the production of white flour, stripping important nutrients from healthy wheat. As various food fads have come and gone, we've called grains a starch and pushed them off the plate, then welcomed them back for their cholesterol-lowering properties. We've embraced them for their fiber, and of late, wrongly feared them for their carbohydrates. We've put bread and pasta at the center of the plate, and then suddenly become downright fearful of gluten. But, as we have wrestled with our definition of the optimum way to eat, the evidence has continued to mount that whole grains are part of it.

Unlike many of the prepared foods that you eat, the consumption of whole grains has been studied in depth, over a long period of time. Whether you eat a carefully planned, health-centered diet or you get your food at the drive-thru, adding whole grains is an easy way to lower your risks of many of the health problems we face today.

You see, the grains that people have been eating for thousands of years were whole grains for most of that time. That means that the bran and germ were intact, whether they were cooked whole or ground into flour. That is the key to the superior nutrition of whole grains. To make white flour or white rice, a whole grain has the bran and germ removed, so most of the minerals, fiber, and vitamins are stripped away. This may make the resulting refined product easier to store and bake or cook with, but it makes it far less nutritious in the bargain.

I know that many of you feel overwhelmed by all the conflicting messages out there. In a world in which billions of dollars are spent on advertising for foods made from refined flour, you have to make the effort to find that loaf of whole wheat bread among the white ones. In a food environment where chemists have used every trick in the book to make junk foods that trigger the same kinds of brain activity as recreational drugs, you have to choose: Will you feed yourself and your family something that provides an addictive thrill but not the nourishment that you need? Or will you pick the whole, real foods that your body truly craves?

Keep it simple. Pick whole.

HEALTH BENEFITS

For our purposes, a serving of grain is $1/2$ cup of cooked whole grain, or about an average slice of 100% whole grain bread. Three servings a day of whole grains is recommended by the USDA.

STROKE

The risk of stroke is reduced by 30 to 36% by consuming three servings per day of whole grain foods.

TYPE 2 DIABETES

Consuming just three servings per day of whole grain foods reduces the risk of developing diabetes by 21 to 30%.

HEART DISEASE

Heart disease risk is reduced by 25 to 28% with three servings per day of whole grains.

WEIGHT MAINTENANCE

In many long-term studies and clinical trials, replacing refined grains with whole ones leads to more weight loss. People who eat whole grains have a lower body mass index (BMI) and a better waist-to-hip ratio. People in these studies who eat three servings of whole grains per day weigh less, have less abdominal fat, and have smaller waists.

INFLAMMATION

Whole grains all contain complex combinations of fiber, anti-inflammatory phytochemicals, and healthy fats. Each unique grain delivers some combination of polysaccharides, saponins, and flavonoids, which work in sync with all the parts of whole grains to cool the fires of inflammation throughout the body.

INTESTINAL WALL PERMEABILITY ("LEAKY GUT")

Many health problems are linked to "leaky gut," a condition in which the digestive tract becomes too permeable and releases proteins and irritants into the bloodstream. Studies have been conducted that show an increase in "trans-epithelial resistance" (a measure of permeability) when subjects switched to a whole grain diet.

COLON CANCER

The fiber in whole grains has been shown to be a potent weapon for reducing risk of colorectal cancer by 20%. With both soluble and insoluble fiber, as well as antioxidants and prebiotics to feed good bacteria, whole grains protect you as you digest them.

ANTIOXIDANTS

Whole grains are a potent source of antioxidants, which have powerful effects in protecting the body. One example of an antioxidant-rich whole grain is popcorn, which has 300 mg of polyphenols per serving, versus 160 g of polyphenols per serving of fruit. Polyphenols are phytochemicals with strong antioxidant effects and are linked to lower risks of cancer and cardiovascular disease. Each grain has its own unique balance of antioxidants, which are absent in refined flours.

PREBIOTICS

Maintaining a healthy balance of beneficial bacteria in the gut is vital to staying well. One of probiotic bacteria's favorite foods is whole grain. Eating yogurt and other fermented foods adds good bacteria to your diet, and the bacteria will thrive in your inner biome if you eat whole grains, beans, and other plant foods for them to help digest.

GLYCEMIC IMPACT

Glycemic impact, more accurately calculated as glycemic load, is the measure of how much a person's blood sugar goes up after consuming a food. Eating lots of high-glycemic-load foods causes elevated blood sugars, which leads to many health problems, including type 2 diabetes, cardiovascular disease, metabolic syndrome, stroke, and depression. A slice of whole wheat bread has a glycemic load of 5; a slice of white bread has a glycemic load of 14. That means that white bread has almost triple the impact on blood sugar. Choosing whole grains helps stabilize blood sugar.

THE PSYCHOLOGY OF "HEALTHY FOOD"

I F YOU ARE INTRODUCING WHOLE GRAIN FOODS TO YOUR FAMILY, IT HELPS TO UNDERSTAND a little psychology. Basically, calling foods "healthy," or "whole grain" may be counterproductive. We have been conditioned for years to expect anything labeled "healthy" to be a less tasty version of a familiar food. If anyone in the group has had a "healthy" food that disappointed, that association may well be the kiss of death for all "healthy" foods that follow. In most cases, everyone will be better off when you emphasize great flavor over fiber and antioxidants. You are up against million-dollar junk-food ad campaigns.

There are two paths to adopting whole grain foods. One group of people will try any food that is touted as healthy and has probably already embraced whole grains. For them, calling a dish whole grain is a selling point and a reason to dive right in. Then there is the second group, those who need to be lead gently along the path. For a little help in bringing your family along, look to Dr. Len Marquart.

Dr. Len Marquart, PhD, RD, associate professor in the Department of Food Science and Nutrition at the University of Minnesota, has been studying this conundrum for many years. In one very telling study, he and his students did a clever experiment with grade school kids, titled: "Gradual incorporation of whole wheat flour into bread products for elementary school children improves whole grain intake."

In the industry, this is referred to as "stealth nutrition."

In the course of a school year, at two different schools, Marquart and his students monitored how many buns and rolls were served to the students, and they also weighed any that were discarded at the end of the meal. In seven gradual increases, the whole grain flour in the buns and rolls was bumped up from 0 to 91%. At one school, white whole wheat flour was used, and at the other, standard red whole wheat flour.

Of course, where the psychology comes in is that the kids were completely in the dark. There were no announcements, no memos to parents. Nobody knew that they were being served something healthy.

The results? The children kept right on eating their bread, blissfully unaware that it was becoming just a little bit whole wheatier every week. Consumption was barely affected. That's right: over the course of the year, kids went from zero whole grain consumption at lunch to one serving, without knowing a thing about it.

The details also give us some clues as to how to slip whole grains into your family's meals.

Here are some tips for using "stealth nutrition" to make whole grains part of your family's favorite foods.

TIP N°1 When whole grain buns were part of the entrée, like a sandwich or sloppy joe, consumption was higher. The more flavorful the filling for the bun, the less aware any testers were of the presence of whole grains.

TIP N°2 Another key to success? White whole wheat flour. This healthy whole grain flour is made from a variety of wheat with a pale bran layer, so the flour looks lighter in color. White whole wheat flour is a versatile ingredient that allows whole grain breads and rolls to look more like the familiar white bread.

TIP N°3 When cooking and baking with whole grains, balance the assertive flavors and textures with a little more spice, seasonings, and snap than you might use with bland white flour or rice. Flavors like chocolate, cinnamon, garlic, herbs, and chiles can all create a harmonious overall taste, while keeping bran and germ from being the predominant element. The chewy textures of whole grains are complemented by lots of other sensations, from a creamy cheese sauce to the pop of peas and crunch of veggies.

TIP N°4 Just like white whole wheat flour, whole wheat pastry flour has a knack for flying under the radar. If you have not used pastry flour, it is made from a kind of soft wheat that is lower in gluten, making a tenderer, pastry-like crumb. It's also finely ground, so it has none of the stone-ground flecks and chew that a hearty whole wheat bread flour imparts.

TIP N°5 Just as you can balance out the hearty flavors of whole wheat, you can use visual distractions to keep your family from becoming too focused on the color shift when baking with whole wheat. Sweet potatoes, carrots, bananas, cinnamon, chocolate, and many other vegetables, fruits, and spices can provide a little cover for your whole wheat flours, enticing diners to enjoy them without probing too deeply. Who looks past a layer of streusel or wonders why a peanut butter cookie or chocolate cake is brown?

You, too, can slip whole grains gradually into favorite foods like pizza and biscuits. Or, you can use whole grains with bold flavors, and your family will be so busy noticing the cinnamon or pumpkin that they will never suspect that you switched out the flours. Just never, ever say that you are taking away a favorite food and serving something "healthy" in its place.

GETTING STARTED

STEP ONE

SO NOW THAT YOU HAVE DECIDED TO MAKE THE EFFORT TO GET WHOLE GRAINS INTO YOUR life, set yourself up to succeed. You can get to that three servings a day almost effortlessly, just by swapping out some foods you normally buy at the grocery store. You don't need to announce this. Once your pantry is filled with tasty and appealing whole foods choices, you and your family will embrace them. They may not even know that certain foods are whole grain, and why tell them? It's just good food.

Your grocery store should carry 100% whole grain versions of these products. Read on for tips on how to read labels to make sure that you are getting true whole grain foods.

BREAD

Swap out white bread for whole wheat bread. If you have a bakery nearby that makes a unique, fresh loaf, it is worth making an extra stop. If your grocer only stocks a few kinds of whole grain bread, speak up. Ask for more whole grain options, and tell your friends to buy them as well.

CEREALS

Switching to whole grain cereals is the easiest swap to make, with many brands of granola and cereal made from all whole grains.

CRACKERS, PRETZELS, AND SNACKS

Crackers have been ahead of the curve on whole grains, with Triscuits, Wheat Thins, and similar products. Look for all your favorite snacks in whole grain versions, from crackers to chips, and always seek out whole grain popcorn.

GRAHAM CRACKERS

Graham crackers were invented by Sylvester Graham as a way to eat more whole wheat. These days, some of them are not 100%, so check that label.

PASTA

Whole wheat pasta has really improved in taste and texture in recent years. Look for 100% whole wheat pasta or branch out in the Asian section with brown rice and buckwheat noodles.

READING LABELS

To be a consistent whole grains consumer, you need to master the art of label reading. Believe it or not, manufacturers sometimes imply that packaged foods are whole grain, when they actually contain just a smidgen. Don't worry, it's not hard to decode. You just need to understand the importance of the order in which things are listed and be aware of a few word games that manufacturers play.

The first ingredient should include the word "whole." Whole wheat flour, whole grain, 100% whole grain. By law, ingredients are listed by weight, so the first ingredient is the one that weighs more than any other ingredient. Calling something "wheat bread" or "100% wheat" means nothing—it can be made with white flour. "Multigrain" is a similarly vague term, and it may mean that a handful of grains have been added to an otherwise white bread. "Stone-ground," "organic," or "natural" doesn't guarantee wholeness unless it is followed by "whole." The word "enriched" is only applied to refined flour. "Made with whole grain" means only that there are some whole grains in there, but it does not tell you how much. When in doubt, look for a Whole Grains Council stamp (there are two types). One stamp says "100% whole grain," and it is your assurance that only whole grains are in the food, no refined grains. The second stamp assures you that a serving of the food delivers at least half a serving of whole grains. These products contain at least half whole grain flour.

Once you have stocked up on whole grain replacements, you can make all your favorite foods with your new options. Is Saturday spaghetti night? Make your usual sauce and serve your whole wheat spaghetti instead—and toss the pasta with the sauce to coat before serving, rather than pouring it on top of the noodles in separate bowls. After-school snack? A box of whole grain graham crackers and a tasty spread and you are good to go. And when the wine and cheese come out, your delicious whole grain crackers and baguette will make the perfect accompaniment.

STEP TWO

Now that your palate is growing accustomed to the heartier, more flavorful whole grain options that you have swapped in, it's time to start cooking with some of the fastest-cooking whole grains. These are weeknight meal savers, mainly because they can be on the table in the same amount of time as white rice.

These grains can be your new go-to for the base of the meal. Serving a stir-fry, thick stew, or curry? Instead of rice, try a whole grain like millet or quinoa. Whole wheat or brown rice couscous is a great alternative for pasta salads and can swap with the orzo in a Greek salad.

It's also perfect for soaking up the flavorful juices of your favorite cut of beef or lamb.

The chart on page 20 has been compiled by speed of cooking. That means that the first listings are the fastest and the last take the longest to cook. Of course, all the grains are wonderful and worth cooking, you just need a little more time in your schedule to cook farro than bulgur.

STEP THREE

Cook some of the longer-cooking grains and start baking with whole grains. This isn't any harder than step two, it just takes a little more time. Brown rice is a bit long cooking, but it's easy to find and easy to introduce to the family, since it's familiar. You may find that the flexibility of boiling a batch of wheat berries is comfortable for you, since you have a long window of time between done and overdone, so you need not worry about messing it up.

Big, fat grains like spelt, barley, and wild rice are juicy and chewy, and may delight your palate most of all.

Baking with whole grains is a great way to really win your family's heart. Who can resist a fragrant, warm muffin just out of the oven? There is nothing quite as appealing as a freshly baked scone, roll, or loaf of bread. If you want to try adding whole grain flours to recipes that you already enjoy, try the stealth method. Start by using one third whole wheat flour instead of white. For tender muffins, scones, or other pastries, use whole wheat pastry flour, and for yeasted breads, use white whole wheat or stone-ground whole wheat flour. Kamut, spelt, and heritage wheats are also delicious options for adding whole wheat with unique flavors. Look to the Switching Whole Wheat Flour for White: Hydration Matters sidebar on page 66 for guidance on the amount of liquid to use when going 100% whole grain.

STRATEGIES FOR MAKING IT EASY (AND SAVING MONEY)

SERVING WHOLE GRAINS CAN BE AN EASY, INEXPENSIVE WAY TO FEED YOUR FAMILY.

BUY BULK. Those bins at the store are a real bargain, and they usually have the price per pound and ounce clearly marked so that you can compare. If you don't have a bulk section at your store, look for large bags of grain that cost less per ounce. Store the extra grain in a dark, cool place in an airtight jar or tub.

COOK AHEAD FOR THE WEEK. This book is full of recipes for using "leftover" grains. That means that you should plan on cooking a large batch every time you cook grains. Make a habit of cooking up a pot of a favorite, or maybe a grain you've never tried before, on the weekend or whenever you have time. Cool at room temperature, then transfer to storage tubs and refrigerate for the week. At the basic level, you can simply stir them in a pan on the stove or microwave them, then serve with milk and fruit for breakfast, on a salad for lunch, or stirred into canned soup for instant dinner.

COOK AHEAD AND FREEZE. If your weeknight meals are made in a hurry, you can save prep time by cooking batches of whole grains and freezing them in portions that work for you. The texture will be best with larger grains, like brown rice, wheat berries, wild rice, etc. Simply cook a few cups of grain, cool completely, then spread loosely on a sheet pan and freeze. Transfer the frozen grain to storage bags or tubs. Make sure you don't pack it so that it freezes solid. You want the grains to be separated. If you think of it the day before you want to serve, thaw the grain in the refrigerator overnight. Or, warm the grain with a few drops of water in the microwave or over low heat on the stove. For optimum texture in delicate grains, put the frozen grain on a piece of parchment in a steamer and steam until thawed and heated through. Don't stir too much or they will break up and become mushy.

STORE BREAKFAST IN JARS. I like to portion out cooked steel-cut oats, porridges, and other grains into 8- and 16-ounce canning jars to freeze. You can even top the porridges with frozen berries and other add-ins so that they are ready to go. The sturdy jars can go into your backpack or bag to thaw as you travel, or you can microwave the jar and add milk, yogurt, or whatever you like.

FREEZE OTHER WHOLE GRAIN FOODS. Those end-of-summer deals at the farmers' market can be made into whole grain soups and then frozen for another day. Great deal on whole wheat bread? Stash it in the freezer and slip individual slices right into the toaster as needed. Same thing with the pancakes and biscuits that you make from your homemade baking mix, or the pizza crusts you make from the recipe in this book.

PASTA-STYLE COOKING

Pasta-style cooking is a method of cooking grains by boiling them in plenty of water like pasta. Some people really like the flexibility of not measuring, just boiling and testing as if you were cooking spaghetti. Drain them in a fine-mesh strainer. I have found that I use this method almost always with bigger grains, like wheat berries, spelt, hulled barley, and wild rice, which often take a long time to cook and absorb varying amounts of water.

Mid-sized grains like brown and pigmented rices can also be cooked this way, as long as you keep close tabs on them for doneness and after draining, put them back in the warm pot and cover, so they can steam for five minutes. This is an important step in the cooking of brown rice, otherwise it may stay crunchy. See sidebar on page 21.

Smaller grains like buckwheat, millet, and quinoa can also be cooked this way, as long as you are careful not to overcook. Drain in a fine-mesh strainer and let stand for a few minutes, then fluff.

Teeny grains like amaranth and teff should really be cooked with the appropriate measure of water and not drained, as much of the grain would be washed away with the water.

SUBSTITUTING GRAINS

If your grocery store has a limited assortment of grains, you may need to substitute something easy to find for something exotic. Depending on your region of the country, brown rice and oats may be your most accessible whole grains. Pearled barley should be around, since people use it in soup, but hulled or hull-less barley may not be. Kasha or buckwheat is also sometimes available if there are people of northern European extraction living in the area. Bulgur is used in Middle Eastern and Mediterranean foods, and you have probably had it in tabouli.

There are also big differences between the cost per pound of various grains, and your budget may not always accommodate imported exotic grains. Grains can always be a budget food, especially if you start comparing prices at all the places you shop. Because they store well, you can stock up when you see them at a good price and save some exciting and slightly pricier grains for special meals. Keep in mind that even the most expensive grains are a bargain compared to many far less nutritious foods.

So, in a pinch, you can always substitute. The chart below should make this easy. Brown rice is quite versatile and can stand in for most grains in salads, soups, and pilafs, as long as you adjust the amount of liquid and the cooking time. For example, if you want to use brown rice instead of millet, you will need the same amount of liquid but 20 to 25 minutes more cooking time. To use brown rice instead of the wheat berries in a salad, cook the same amount of rice but use the correct ratio of liquid and cook for 40 to 45 minutes, then chill.

GRAIN COOKING CHART

Let me share one important fact: You can cook grains in different ways to achieve different textures. Toasting the grain beforehand keeps it a little firmer, as well as giving it a nutty flavor. Using the minimum amount of water keeps the grain more firm and separate, while cooking it in more water will make it softer in most cases. Grains like buckwheat, millet, and brown rice can be cooked to a porridge consistency with more liquids and more time. Grains like wheat berries and whole rye will stay whole and separate for a long time, no matter how much liquid you cook them in, so if you add them to a porridge they will be a crunchy, separate part of the mix.

GRAIN	RATIO OF LIQUID TO GRAIN IN CUPS	COOKING TIME AND YIELD
Whole wheat couscous	1½ to 1 (or soak for 1 hour in cold water)	5 minutes steaming Makes 2½ cups
Bulgur	1½ to 1 (or soak for 2 hours in cold water)	10 minutes steaming Makes 3 cups
Quinoa	1¼–1½ to 1	15 minutes Makes 3 cups
Kañiwa	2 to 1	15 minutes Makes 2 cups
Millet	2–2½ to 1	25 minutes Makes 2½ to 3 cups
Buckwheat groats	1½–2 to 1	15 to 20 minutes Makes 3 to 4 cups
Teff	3 to 1	20 minutes Makes 2½ cups
Amaranth	2½–3 to 1	25 minutes
"Green wheat" freekeh (available whole or cracked)	2½ to 1	Whole: 40 to 45 minutes Cracked: 25 to 30 minutes Makes 3 cups
Short-grain brown rice	2 to 1	40 to 45 minutes Makes 3 cups
Long-grain brown rice	1½–2 to 1	40 to 45 minutes Makes 3 cups
Black and red rice	There are different varieties, check the package directions; if you have black rice with no package, start with 1½ cups water to 1 cup rice and cook for 25 minutes. Himalayan red rice is as short as 15 minutes. If you have red rice with no package, start with 1¾ cups water to 1 cup rice and cook for 20 minutes.	
Pearled barley	2 to 1	40 minutes Makes 3 cups
Whole, hulled, or hull-less barley, purple or black	Soaking and "pasta-style" cooking recommended 2½ to 1 / 1½ to 1	1 hour or more Makes 3½ cups
Steel-cut oats	4 to 1	30 minutes Makes 3 cups
Steel-cut oats	4 to 1	in the slow cooker on low 4½ to 5 hours Makes 3 cups
Whole oat groats	2–3 to 1	1 hour Makes 3 cups
Whole wheat, farro, kamut, and rye berries	Soaking and "pasta-style" cooking recommended 3 to 1	45 minutes to 1 hour Makes 3 cups

SOAKING GRAINS

There are three reasons to soak grains.

The first, and most direct, is soaking bulgur or whole wheat couscous as a replacement for cooking it. Using a one-to-one water-to-grain ratio, you can simply pour cold water over bulgur or whole wheat couscous, cover, and refrigerate for two hours or overnight. If there is any excess water, drain and squeeze the grains gently. Bulgur comes in a variety of sizes, but the common medium-grain bulgur will rehydrate in about two hours. Whole wheat couscous rehydrates in about an hour.

A second reason to soak grains is to shave off cooking time and to make the grains more digestible. Long-cooking grains, like brown rice or wheat berries, will cook in about five minutes less. The soaking of grains for enhanced digestibility is a little more controversial. All grains, and many plant foods, contain a few undesirable natural chemicals along with the desirable ones. In grains, something called phytic acid resides in the bran layer. This acid can bind with the calcium, iron, and zinc in the grain and make them hard to absorb. For many years, whole foods advocates recommended soaking all grains and flours before eating, to remove this acid. The science behind this has become murkier, and we now know that phytic acid is an antioxidant. If you are concerned about getting the full measure of nutrients from grains, soak them overnight, then drain and cook, setting the timer five minutes earlier than directed. For breads, overnight soaks and ferments, as well as sourdoughs, break down the phytic acid and make the grains more digestible and absorbable.

A third reason to soak grains is to sprout them. Sprouting also changes the chemistry of a grain, decreasing some chemicals that make them hard to digest and slightly increasing some nutrients. Soaking grains like wheat berries until a little white sprout appears, then cooking them, will make slightly softer grains with a sweeter flavor.

BROWN RICE AND ARSENIC

You may have heard about it in the news in 2012, when the story on arsenic in brown rice was published in *Consumer Reports*. Overnight, a food we all associated with healthy eating was under suspicion. In response, rice growers and USDA scientists have been testing and monitoring the levels of organic and inorganic arsenic in brown rice.

It turns out that the rice plant needs silica to form its healthy bran layer, but if it is grown in soil with arsenic present, it will use that in silica's place. Organic arsenic occurs naturally in some soils, and inorganic arsenic (considered more hazardous to health) has also been used in pesticides, along with occasionally being fed to chickens, whose manure is used as fertilizer. That means that some brown rice, depending on the soil where it is grown, will have higher levels of organic arsenic than are considered healthy. Arsenic is a known carcinogen, but not enough is known to be sure exactly what level of consumption is safe.

As of 2014, the highest levels of arsenic were in brown rice grown in Arkansas, Louisiana, and Texas. California-grown rice had 38 percent less arsenic than those. Rice from India and

Pakistan is also lower in arsenic. *Consumer Reports*, based on their ongoing research, recommends that adults consume only ½ cup per week of uncooked brown rice (about 1½ cups cooked), and children should only eat a little more than half of that.

To continue enjoying the health benefits of brown rice, buy from the regions with the lowest levels of arsenic. You can also reduce the arsenic levels by 10 to 30 percent by washing the rice until the water runs clear. Cooking rice "pasta-style" in lots of boiling water reduced the arsenic by 25 to 45 percent, but that method also reduces the B vitamins that make it so healthful.

So, try black or red rice, or any of the grains in the book—they are all safe. The *Consumer Reports* website posts their findings, brand by brand, so you can check there to see which brown rice to buy. And it's still fine to eat brown rice; we just need to mix it up a little!

APPLIANCES: RICE COOKERS, SLOW COOKERS, AND PRESSURE COOKERS

Let it be said, you can cook whole grains with nothing but a pot and some heat. Just ask the Ojibwe and Chippewa, who cooked wild rice over a fire thousands of years ago. But you might find that a few modern appliances will make whole grains easier to celebrate in your busy life.

The electric rice cooker is a handy tool for people who want to set it and forget it. Today's cookers are engineered to cook rice perfectly and can easily be used to cook other whole grains as well. Buy one with a brown rice setting, and you may find that the rice that comes out is the best you have ever had. The benefit of using the cooker is that you can put your grains, water, or other flavorful liquids, and even vegetables and spices, in the cooker, close the lid, and go about your business. The cooker does the rest and when the grain is done, it switches to "keep warm" mode to hold it for you. I use mine to make "one pot" meals, with veggies, proteins, and grains all cooking in a flavorful liquid.

Even more hands-off than the rice cooker is the slow cooker, which does a gentle job of slowly cooking your grains, soups, and other foods. I use a one-quart cooker to make porridges and steel-cut oats while I'm around the house or running errands. A larger cooker is a great way to make up big batches of grains and doubles to simmer soups and stews. The slowness of the cooker means that you can ignore it, but very few grains can cook for the eight hours that you might need them to cook while at work or sleeping.

The pressure cooker is one of the most effective tools for cooking whole grains and, in this country, one that is not used enough. These amazing cookers shave valuable minutes from your whole grain preparation time and do a great job of thoroughly cooking grains.

If you have memories of Grandma's pressure cooker exploding and spraying pea soup everywhere, it's time that you met today's pressure cooker. Safe, well-engineered pressure cookers now have pressure release and easy-to-use regulating valves. They come in small, medium, and large, for all your needs. A four- or six-quart cooker will do a good job of cooking small amounts of grain and will be more versatile in your kitchen. Once you've delved into cooking brown rice in the pressure cooker, you can use it to speedily prepare dried beans, vegetables, stews, and even whole roasts and chickens.

GLOSSARY OF GRAINS AND FLOURS

AMARANTH

Technically not a grain but a pseudograin from the Goosefoot family, amaranth was the staple food of the Aztecs. It's incredibly nutritious, with lots of protein, calcium, and even essential fatty acids. It's also gluten-free. Amaranth, like teff, is tiny, and it can't really be cooked to be separate and fluffy; it tends more toward turning into porridge or polenta. The teeny seeds can be popped, as they are in Mexico, where they are made into a sweet treat called *alegria*. For a crunchy addition to baked goods, first soak the seeds in water or simply add them raw.

BARLEY

Barley is one of the best grains for lowering cholesterol. It contains a remarkably effective cholesterol-cleansing starch called beta-glucan, the same one that is in oats. It also contains a small amount of gluten. Whole, unhulled barley is somewhat confusingly referred to as "hull-less" barley or even "naked barley." This is because the standard variety of barley has a clingy, hard-to-remove hull and is usually "pearled," a process that scrapes off not just the hull but also the underlying bran layer. Hull-less barley still has its bran layer and comes in purple and black versions.

BUCKWHEAT

Buckwheat is not related to wheat and contains no gluten. The earthy, nutty-tasting grain is most often ground for flour, which we see most commonly in pancakes. Buckwheat is more than just a pancake flour, however. The groats make delicious pilafs, burgers, and hot cereals. Buckwheat is high in minerals and in a particularly potent anti-inflammatory chemical called rutin.

BULGUR

Bulgur is whole wheat that has been parboiled, dried, and chipped into granules of different sizes. Parboiling makes it cook more quickly, and you can even soak it in cold water to rehydrate. The standard bulgur that you will find in American stores is classified as medium grain, but if you seek out a Middle Eastern grocery, you will find much smaller grades of bulgur, each with its own traditional use. Tiny bulgur is used in dishes like kibbeh or certain salads. The process of parboiling the grain actually drives the nutrients deeper into the grain, making it a very nutritious food.

COUSCOUS

Couscous may look like a whole grain, but it's really a form of pasta, made from flour. Whole wheat or brown rice couscous, however, is also available. They are very quick cooking and can even be rehydrated by soaking in cold water. In North Africa, where couscous originated, millet was the original grain that was ground and shaped into couscous, but they switched over to using durum wheat in the twentieth century. In some regions barley is used to make couscous. There is also a larger, rounder version referred to as "pearl" or "Israeli" couscous, which is sometimes made with whole wheat flour and has to be boiled like pasta.

FONIO

A staple food in Senegal, fonio is hard to find in the United States. It's a shame, since it is a very nutritious, exciting grain. High in complete protein, iron, and other minerals, fonio is at the base of most traditional Senegalese meals, where a large bowl of cooked fonio is at the table and curries and vegetables are eaten with it. The grains are tiny, smaller than amaranth or teff, making them difficult to clean, so it is best to rinse them in a fine-mesh strainer before cooking.

FREEKEH

Green wheat freekeh is similar to bulgur, although it is made from immature (green) wheat and the grain is roasted rather than parboiled. The original process involved piling up the soft, immature wheat, still on the stalk, and setting it on fire to remove the chaff and roast the grains. Because the wheat was still moist inside, it didn't burn. Now, the grain is roasted instead of fire-roasted. This gives freekeh a smoky, toasty flavor. It is then rubbed and cleaned and dried whole or broken into pieces. It's relatively high in protein and has the same zinc, calcium, and iron that wheat has.

KAÑIWA

Closely related to quinoa, kañiwa has grains half the size of its popular relative. It's also lacking in the bitter saponins that coat quinoa, so it doesn't need to be washed, and it has a naturally sweet, nutty flavor. Kañiwa, like quinoa, is high in protein, fiber, iron, and calcium, and it cooks quickly. Because of its small size, it is more likely to be used in porridges than salads. With its deep, sweet flavor and delicate crunch, it's kind of like a cross between teff and quinoa. As of this writing, kañiwa is not easy to find in stores, but it should grow in popularity and become more available.

MILLET

The golden grains of millet are most often seen in birdseed mixes, but millet really deserves a second look in the kitchen. Sweet and mild, this yellow grain is gluten-free and has none of the branny flavors that can make whole grains a challenge. Millet is also very versatile, capable of cooking up firm and separate or, with more liquid, making a sticky polenta or porridge. Millet is a standout for containing high levels of magnesium, copper, phosphorus, and manganese, all of which are very protective of your health.

OATS

Everyone loves oats, don't they? As a hot cereal or in a cookie or bar, oats have been with us since we were kids. Oats are a sweet, mild grain that has the distinction of being sold in rolled form, making it so easy to use. Just about any grain can be rolled, but for some reason, oats are the one we get. Oats are famous for containing beta-glucans and other starches that sweep cholesterol from the body. They are very high in manganese and molybdenum, and high in copper, biotin, B1, and zinc. Oats are loaded with fiber, too. Gluten-free oats are available, which are guaranteed to have been grown and processed in a gluten-free environment.

QUINOA

This ancient grain that was the staple food for the Inca people was also central to religious ceremonies. Unfortunately, growing quinoa was outlawed after the Spanish took over, to hasten the Westernization of the culture. Quinoa was thought to be lost to us until scientists found it growing wild. It's now one of the most popular whole grains because of its nutty flavor, quick cooking time, and high protein and calcium content. Quinoa is also gluten-free and very digestible. The quinoa plant deters pests by producing bitter, soapy-tasting compounds called saponins, which coat the seeds as they grow. You will see recipes that instruct you to carefully rinse the grain to remove these, but these days, manufacturers have gotten smart and started washing the grain before packaging.

RICE

Whole grain rices are a world unto themselves, encompassing the "pigmented" rices in black, red, purple, and many shades in between. They also come in different lengths—long, medium, and short—and may even be called "glutinous," although they never contain gluten. Long-grain rice and short-grain rice contain two kinds of starch, called amylose and amylopectin. The firmer of these two starches, amylose, which also absorbs more water, is higher in long-grain rice. The softer, more gelatinous starch, amylopectin, is higher in short-grain rice. In general, the bran layer that surrounds each rice grain keeps the inner starches well contained. Short-grain and medium-grain rices in their polished, white forms, often used for risotto and sushi, will exude starches as they cook, but to achieve the same effect with a whole grain rice, you need to stir vigorously enough to break the starches free.

Brown rice is a very good source of manganese, selenium, copper, phosphorous, and B3. Rice is gluten-free and high in fiber.

RYE

Rye is a grain that is made into flour for baking, far more often than it is sold in whole groat form. Rolled rye can sometimes be found as well. Rye is native to northern Europe and Russia, where it grows readily in challenging conditions. It's closely related to wheat and barley and also contains gluten, but not very much. Whole rye is a spicy, deeply flavorful grain, and it makes a good addition to meaty stews and strongly flavored pilafs and vegetarian dishes. Rye is uniquely high in a form of soluble fiber that has a high satiety factor, making it an excellent food to keep you full when on a weight-loss plan. Like many grains, it is high in manganese, phosphorus, copper, pantothenic acid, and magnesium.

TEFF

Teff is one of the tiny grains, native to North Africa, that once fed an entire culture. The hardy grass thrives in poor soil and produces seeds in a short amount of time, making it a good crop for people on the move. It's also high in protein, calcium, iron, and fiber. The most well known use for teff is to make *injera*, a fermented pancake-like flatbread. If you have ever eaten at a North African restaurant in which the "plate" was a pillowy sourdough pancake, you have had *injera*. Whole grain teff cooks up like a porridge, with a delightful crunch from all the tiny little seeds. The grains can be used whole in baking or soaked and added to batters, or you can use the soft grain in hot cereals, soups, and polentas. Teff is gluten-free, and the flour is a beautiful deep brown, with a hint of cocoa flavor.

BREAKFAST

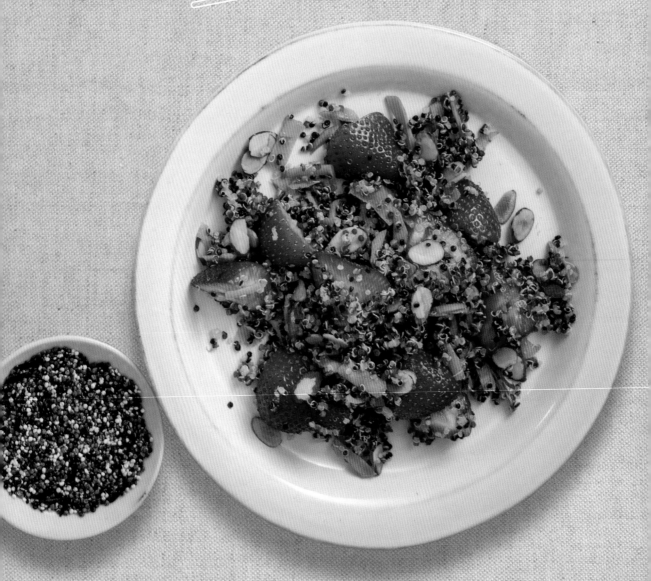

OVERNIGHT OAT SOAK
WITH POMEGRANATE, BERRIES, AND NUTS

Who has time to stir a pot of oats on the stove? All you need is a little planning, and you can let your oats soak peacefully in the refrigerator overnight. Taking inspiration from Swiss muesli, which is soaked overnight, this easy breakfast will become your go-to. This version infuses the oats with antioxidant-rich pomegranate juice, and you can throw in frozen or dried fruit, too.

SERVES 4

1 cup pomegranate juice
½ cup plain yogurt or kefir
1½ cups rolled oats or rolled barley
1 cup frozen berries, or ½ cup dried fruit
½ cup nuts, toasted

In a 1-quart storage bowl or tub, stir together the juice and the yogurt. Stir in the oats and fruit. Cover tightly and refrigerate overnight, or for at least 8 hours. Sprinkle with the nuts just before serving so the nuts will stay crunchy.

Stir and serve cold, or microwave for 2 minutes per bowl.

Keeps for 1 week, tightly covered, in the refrigerator.

TOASTING AND SAUTÉING GRAINS

There is a simple trick that can add a flavor boost to your everyday whole grain cookery. Your grains are already a little nutty tasting, and you can really bring that flavor forward by simply dry-toasting or sautéing them before cooking.

To dry-toast, just measure your uncooked grains into a dry pan, place over medium-high heat, and swirl the pan until the grains crackle and become fragrant. Be careful that you don't burn them. Have water or stock ready to add to the pan so that you can stop the toasting. Of course, when you add the liquid to the hot pan it will bubble up rather dramatically, so first take the pan off the heat and have the lid ready to cover the pan.

To sauté, just heat a little oil or butter in a pan over medium heat and sauté the uncooked grains. Add a little garlic or spice, and you get even more flavor. For extra-special steel-cut oats, try sautéing them in brown butter. Just heat a tablespoon or two of unsalted butter over medium heat until the butter begins to turn brown and little brown flecks appear. It will smell nutty, not burned. Add the steel-cut oats, stir to coat, and cook for a couple of minutes until slightly toasted. Then add your liquid and proceed.

BOIL-AND-LEAVE STEEL-CUT OATS

Steel-cut oats are famous for their cholesterol-lowering, hunger-satisfying fiber. You can skip the stovetop time by giving them a boiling start, then leaving them to soak. After an hour or more, just bring them back to a boil and they will be wonderfully tender and ready to embellish with your favorite fruit, sweeteners, and spice.

SERVES 4

1 cup steel-cut oats
4 cups water
Pinch of salt

Put the oats in a 2-quart pot, preferably one with a heavy bottom. Place over high heat and swirl the oats until they smell toasty, about 3 minutes. Take off the heat and carefully pour in the water. It will bubble up when it hits the hot pan, so be careful.

Add the salt and put back over high heat. Bring to a full boil.

Turn off the heat and cover. Let stand at room temperature for at least an hour or overnight.

To serve, place over high heat and bring back to a boil, then stir for 5 minutes.

Serve hot, with toppings, or transfer to a storage tub and reheat as needed.

Keeps for 1 week, tightly covered, in the refrigerator.

QUICK STOVETOP GRANOLA

I love a good, slow-baked granola, but sometimes there isn't time. That's when this version saves the day! Instead of baking the oats, just pan-toast them, and when the oats are fragrant and hot, swirl in the remaining ingredients. The sugar or maple syrup will melt into the oats, providing a gentle, slightly caramelized sweetness. The whole process goes fast, so be ready with a large bowl to dump the granola into before it burns.

SERVES 4

½ cup packed light brown sugar, or ¼ cup maple syrup

1 teaspoon cinnamon

¼ teaspoon salt

2 cups rolled oats

½ cup walnuts, pecans, or whole almonds

1 tablespoon unsalted butter or canola oil

Dried fruit (optional)

In a cup, stir together the brown sugar, cinnamon, and salt and reserve. (If using maple syrup, measure it out but do not combine with the cinnamon and salt mixture). Have a large bowl ready for transferring the hot granola out of the pan.

In a large sauté pan, combine the oats and nuts. Over medium heat, swirl and stir the mixture until it becomes hot to the touch, about 5 minutes. Keep the oats moving in the pan so that they don't burn. Keep cooking until the oats are lightly golden and toasty smelling. Toss in the butter and stir rapidly to coat the grains, then add the sugar mixture or the maple syrup and the cinnamon and salt. Turn the heat down to low, stirring and scraping, to coat the oats as the sugar melts.

Continue to stir and mix. Take off the heat once the oats are coated in sugar (or, if you are using maple syrup, once the granola looks dry) and quickly scrape into the large bowl. Let cool for at least 5 minutes before serving, as it will be hot. Stir in the fruit, if desired.

Let cool completely and transfer to a storage tub or resealable plastic bags.

Keeps for 10 days, tightly covered, at room temperature.

SUPER-CHUNKY
SWEET CHERRY-ALMOND GRANOLA

If you have ever eaten granola with your fingers, picking out the glistening clusters and leaving the rest behind, this granola is for you. This is dessert or snack granola that you can eat one sweet, crunchy chunk at a time.

SERVES 12

4 cups rolled oats
1 cup whole almonds, coarsely chopped
1 teaspoon coarse salt
1 tablespoon cinnamon
½ cup canola oil
½ cup honey
½ cup packed light brown sugar
1 teaspoon vanilla extract
1 cup dried sweet cherries

Preheat the oven to 350°F.

In a large bowl, stir together the oats, almonds, salt, and cinnamon.

In a medium bowl, stir together the oil, honey, brown sugar, and vanilla. Pour over the oat mixture and mix well.

Line a rimmed baking sheet with parchment paper. Spread the oat mixture over the paper in a thick, even layer.

Bake for 20 minutes, stir, then bake for 20 minutes more. The granola will be soft and flexible. Stir in the cherries. Use your spatula to press the granola flat in the pan, forming a compressed layer. Put back in the oven for 10 minutes.

Let cool in the pan on a rack. When completely cool, break into large chunks and store in jars or tubs.

Keeps for 10 days, tightly covered, at room temperature.

DAILY WALNUT-RAISIN OLIVE OIL GRANOLA

Drop that packaged cereal and start making this tasty granola, kissed with healthy olive oil and endlessly variable. Prefer pecans or almonds? Currants or dates? It's all good in this wonderfully chewy, satisfying breakfast in a bowl. This is a classic "loose" granola, with fewer big chunks and lots of chewy oat flavor.

SERVES 6

¼ cup extra-virgin olive oil, plus more for the pan

4 cups rolled oats

1 large orange, zested and juiced

½ teaspoon salt

½ cup maple syrup

1 cup walnuts, coarsely chopped

1 cup raisins

Preheat the oven to 325°F. Lightly oil a large rimmed sheet pan. In a large bowl, combine the oats, orange zest, and salt. In a medium bowl, measure ¼ cup of the juice from the orange (save any extra for another use). Stir in the olive oil and maple syrup, then pour the mixture over the oats. Stir and toss the oats to coat with the maple mixture, then stir in the walnuts. Spread on the prepared pan.

Bake for 20 minutes, then stir. Return the pan to the oven and repeat two more times, for a total baking time of 1 hour.

Stir in the raisins and let cool in the pan on a rack. Let cool completely before transferring to an airtight container.

Keeps for 10 days, tightly covered, at room temperature.

DATE *AND* GRAIN ENERGY BARS

There are all sorts of "energy" products out there with weird refined sweeteners and protein isolates. Get back to nature with the quick energy of dried fruit and the slow-burning carbs of whole grains. A tasty protein boost from nut butter makes these a perfect packable snack for long bike rides or hikes.

SERVES 16

Canola oil, for the pan

¾ cup rolled oats, divided

2 cups (10 ounces) soft pitted dates

2 cups (10 ounces) dried apricots or cherries

¼ cup almond butter

1 teaspoon vanilla extract

½ teaspoon almond extract

1 tablespoon freshly grated lemon zest

2 tablespoons freshly squeezed lemon juice

1½ cups cooked millet or other grain (½ cup uncooked)

2 tablespoons whole wheat pastry flour

Oil an 8-inch square pan, then sprinkle ¼ cup of the oats in the pan. In a food processor, combine ¼ cup oats, the dates, apricots, almond butter, vanilla, almond extract, lemon zest, and lemon juice. Pulse the processor to coarsely purée the fruit and mix well. Break up the mixture if it has formed a ball in the processor bowl and sprinkle the cooked grain and flour into the bowl. Pulse to mix but not further purée.

Scrape out into a bowl to finish mixing with your hands, if necessary. Place large dollops of the mixture into the prepared pan. Spread and flatten the mixture with a spatula to make an even layer. Sprinkle with the remaining ¼ cup oats and chill.

Cut the chilled bars 4 x 4 to make 16 bars. Transfer to an airtight container.

Keeps for 2 weeks, tightly covered, in the refrigerator.

THREE SUPER SMOOTHIES

Smoothies are everywhere, and for good reason. Slipping spinach, berries, whole grains, and other healthy foods into a slurpable, shake-like treat is brilliant. I like to use fruit that is fully frozen so the resulting texture is smooth and creamy. Here are two smoothies with cooked grain blended right in, and one smoothie that forms a tasty moat for an island of crunchy granola.

BLUEBERRY GREEN SMOOTHIE WITH LEFTOVER GRAIN

SERVES 2

4 cups (4 ounces) fresh baby spinach

1 medium frozen banana

1 cup coconut water, kefir, or almond milk

2 cups (8 ounces) frozen blueberries

½ cup cooked millet, brown rice, oats, or amaranth

In a blender, combine the ingredients in order, then blend. Purée until very smooth and thick, stopping to scrape down as necessary. Using fully frozen berries and bananas will create a very thick, milkshake consistency.

Serve immediately.

STRAWBERRY-BANANA QUINOA SMOOTHIE

SERVES 2

2 cups frozen strawberries

1 cup cooked quinoa

1 cup plain kefir or yogurt

1 medium frozen banana

Combine all the ingredients in a blender and process to make a thick shake.

Serve immediately.

GRANOLA ISLAND SMOOTHIE

SERVES 2

2 cups (2 ounces) fresh spinach

1 cup frozen strawberries

½ cup nonfat vanilla yogurt

½ cup pomegranate juice

½ cup granola (see recipes on pages 31-33)

In the following order, put the spinach, strawberries, yogurt, and pomegranate juice in a blender. Purée until very smooth.

Divide the smoothie between two cereal bowls and pile half of the granola in the middle of each bowl.

Serve immediately.

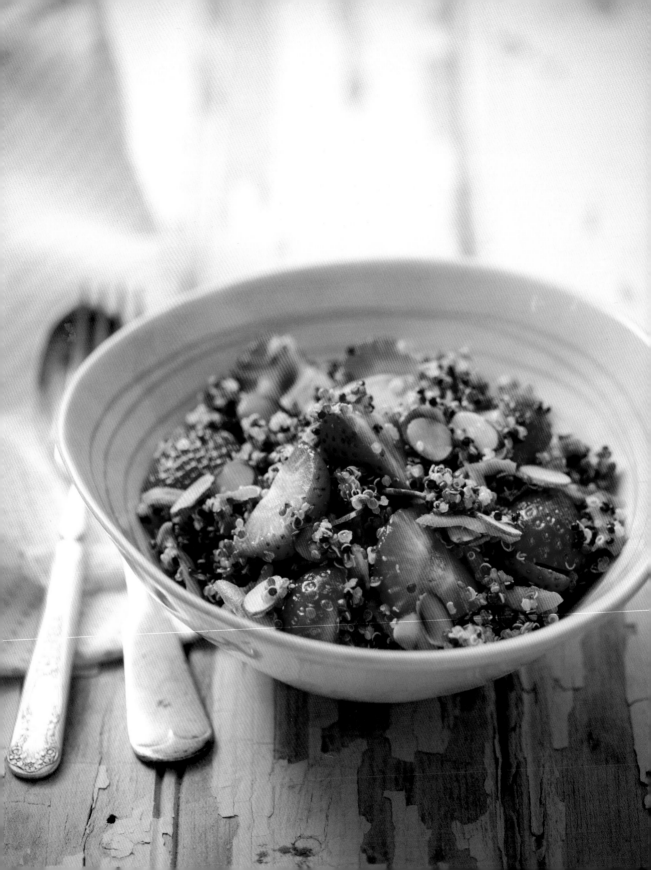

LEMON-STRAWBERRY
QUINOA BREAKFAST SALAD

Grain salads are not just for picnics and lunchboxes! When summer comes, a cool, grainy breakfast salad is a great way to start the day. Quinoa and juicy berries are light and fresh with lemon and will fuel your morning adventures in a delightful way.

SERVES 4

3 cups cooked quinoa (1 cup uncooked)
1 pound fresh strawberries, halved
1 cup shredded carrot
3 tablespoons honey
3 tablespoons freshly squeezed lemon juice
1 tablespoon canola oil
½ teaspoon salt
½ cup sliced almonds, toasted

Put the cooked quinoa in a large bowl. Add the strawberries and carrot. In a cup, stir together the honey, lemon, canola oil, and salt, then pour over the quinoa and toss to coat.

Chill for up to 3 days. Serve topped with sliced almonds.

FARRO WITH CLEMENTINES *AND* YOGURT DRESSING

Cook up some crunchy, hearty farro, and this salad practically makes itself. You can use canned clementines or mandarin oranges, and the simple yogurt dressing comes together in a snap. You can make it the night before and pack it the next morning for your busy day.

SERVES 4

4 cups water

1 cup farro or other grain

6 small clementines or mandarin oranges

½ cup plain yogurt

1 tablespoon freshly squeezed lemon juice

¼ cup honey

½ cup crystallized ginger, chopped

¼ cup chopped fresh parsley

In a 1-quart pot, bring the water to a boil and add the farro. Reduce the heat to a vigorous simmer and cook for 40 minutes or more, until tender. Drain and let cool to room temperature.

Peel and section the clementines and put in a large bowl. Add the cooled farro. In a cup, stir together the yogurt, lemon, and honey and pour over the farro mixture. Add the crystallized ginger and parsley and toss to mix.

Serve at room temperature or chill for up to 1 week before serving.

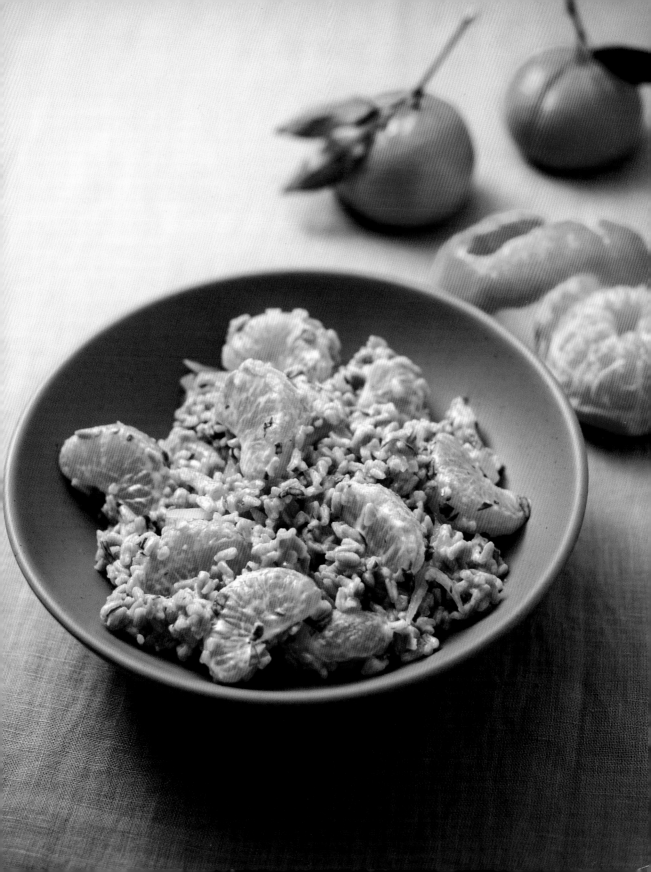

LEFTOVER-GRAIN OMELETS *AND* SCRAMBLES

Everybody is looking for a quick breakfast with some extra protein, and this is a perfect solution. Eggs are quick to cook, and that big batch of healthy whole grains provides a satisfying, chewy filling that will start your day out right.

SERVES 2

4 large eggs
¼ teaspoon salt, divided
1 tablespoon extra-virgin olive oil, divided
½ cup chopped onion
1 medium Roma tomato, diced
1 cup chopped vegetables, such as cauliflower, broccoli, or kale
3 garlic cloves, minced
½ cup cooked grain
¼ cup (1 ounce) shredded cheese

Whisk the eggs and half of the salt in a small bowl and set aside. In a large sauté pan, heat 2 teaspoons of the olive oil and add the onion and tomato. If you are using firm veggies like cauliflower, add that too. Sauté until the onions are soft and golden. If the veggies are still crisp when pierced with a knife, cover the pan and cook on low for 3 minutes. Add leafy greens, if using, and cook for about 2 minutes. Add the garlic and remaining salt and stir for a minute. Stir in the cooked grain.

If you are doing a scramble, push the grain mixture to one side and pour in the whisked eggs. Scramble them over medium heat, stirring in the grain mixture as they start to set. When the eggs are cooked, remove the pan from the heat and sprinkle with cheese. Let sit for 1 minute, or until the cheese melts, then serve.

For an omelet, set the grain mixture aside. In a medium (10-inch) sauté pan or cast-iron pan over high heat, pour a teaspoon of the olive oil and smear it around with your spatula to coat the pan. Whisk the eggs vigorously for a minute, then pour in the pan. Reduce the heat to medium and cook until the eggs are firm and browned on the bottom, with only a thin layer of soft egg on top.

Reheat the grain mixture and stir in the cheese, then spread the mixture on half of the omelet. Fold the eggs over the grain mixture and cook for a couple of minutes, just to melt the cheese and finish cooking that top layer of egg.

Slide the omelet onto a plate, then carefully cut in half and transfer half to another plate. Serve hot.

GRILLED STEEL-CUT OAT SLABS
WITH SAUTÉED APPLES

Once you have the oats cooked and chilled in the pan, you can grill these slabs at any time of the day! If you tire of eating your oats with a spoon, try them this way and enjoy them with a fork. If an apple a day keeps the doctor away, adding an apple to your cholesterol-fighting oats can only add insurance.

SERVES 4

OATS

Canola oil, for the pans

$2\frac{1}{2}$ cups water

$\frac{3}{4}$ cup steel-cut oats

$\frac{1}{2}$ cup rolled oats

2 tablespoons packed light brown sugar

$\frac{1}{4}$ teaspoon salt

APPLES

2 tablespoons unsalted butter

4 medium Granny Smith apples, peeled and sliced

$\frac{1}{4}$ cup packed light brown sugar

1 teaspoon cinnamon

Vanilla yogurt (optional)

Lightly oil an $8\frac{1}{2}$ x $4\frac{1}{2}$-inch loaf pan. In a 2-quart pot, combine the water, steel-cut oats, rolled oats, brown sugar, and salt. Bring to a boil, then cover tightly and reduce the heat to low. Cook for 20 minutes. Uncover and stir thoroughly, then take off the heat and let stand, covered, for 10 minutes. Stir again.

Scrape the oats into the loaf pan and cool on a rack. Cover with plastic wrap and chill until completely cold and firm.

Before serving, let the oats in the loaf pan come to room temperature. Meanwhile, prepare the apples. Melt the butter in a large sauté pan and add the sliced apples. Raise the heat to medium high and stir the apples until they are softened and a little browned in spots, 5 to 7 minutes. When the apples are tender, sprinkle in the brown sugar and cinnamon. Stir until the sugar is melted. Take off the heat and keep warm.

For the oats, oil and heat a cast-iron grill pan or skillet over medium-high heat. Slice the oat loaf into 8 pieces and place them in the hot pan. Cook each side for about 2 minutes, or until browned. Serve 2 slices per plate and top with a quarter of the sautéed apples. Serve with yogurt, if desired.

The chilled pan of oats and the sautéed apples keep for 1 week, tightly covered, in the refrigerator.

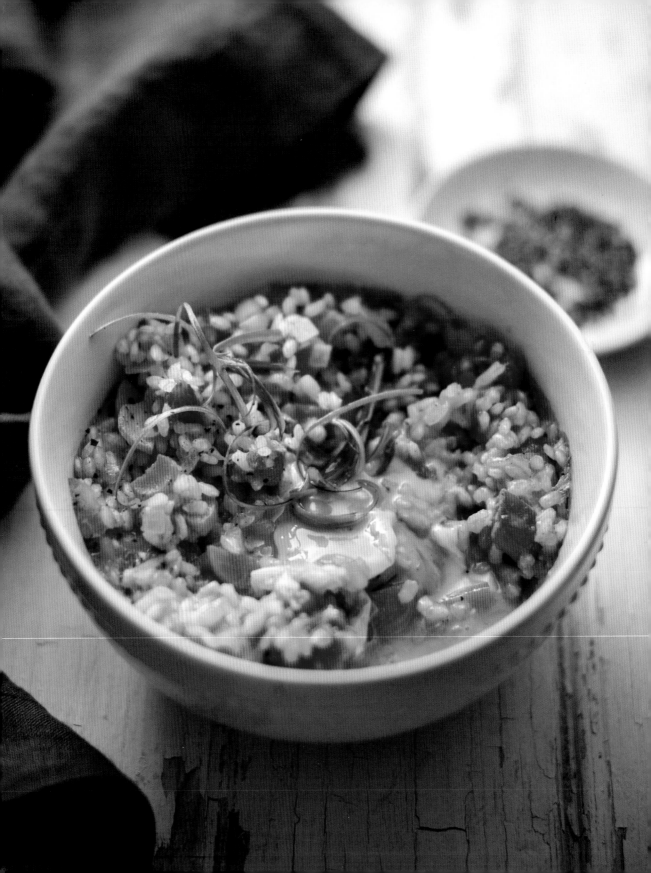

ASIAN BREAKFAST BOWLS

Outside of the good old USA, breakfast isn't always about donuts and cereal from a box. Believe it or not, bowls of rice or other grains can be topped with all sorts of delicious, not-so-sweet foods. Take a break from the same old breakfast and try a rice bowl with some Asian flair—you might just find that a shot of hot sauce is better than coffee!

JAPANESE BREAKFAST BOWL

SERVES 1

1 cup cooked quinoa, rice, or other grain

2 large eggs, whisked

1 teaspoon soy sauce

1/4 cup granulated sugar

1 scallion, sliced on a diagonal (white and green parts)

1/2 teaspoon canola oil

1 cup watercress leaves or fresh baby spinach leaves

2 ounces lox or smoked salmon

1 or 2 pinches rehydrated wakame seaweed or sauerkraut (optional)

If using leftover grain, warm the cooked grain and set aside in a serving bowl.

In a medium bowl, whisk the eggs, soy sauce, sugar, and scallion. Heat a small skillet over medium heat, then coat the pan with the canola oil. Pour in the egg mixture and scramble the eggs, using a spatula to scrape the cooked eggs and turn the mixture.

Top the grain in the bowl with the watercress and place the hot eggs on top, wilting the leaves slightly. Place the lox to one side of the bowl. Tuck a few spoonfuls of seaweed or kraut along the other side of the bowl, if desired, and serve.

EGG CURRY BREAKFAST BOWL

SERVES 4

1/2 cup coconut milk

1 medium carrot, chopped

1/2 cup chopped onion

1 tablespoon chopped fresh ginger

2 teaspoons curry powder

1 teaspoon packed light brown sugar

1/2 teaspoon salt

1 (15-ounce) can diced tomatoes

1 1/2 cups cooked brown rice or other grain

4 large eggs, or 8 ounces soft tofu, cubed

2 scallions, sliced lengthwise (white and green parts)

Preheat the oven to 400°F with the bottom rack positioned at the lowest level.

In a large nonstick skillet, heat the coconut milk and add the carrot, onion, and ginger. Stir over medium heat until the carrot is softened and the coconut milk is thick.

Stir in the curry powder, brown sugar, salt, and tomatoes and mix well. Bring to a boil and stir in the rice.

Divide the rice among 4 ovenproof ramekins or bowls and make a depression in the center of each. Crack an egg into each depression (or add tofu). Bake for 20 to 25 minutes, to your desired level of doneness. (You may want a firmer yolk or a runny one; a runny yolk will act as a sauce.)

Top with scallions and serve immediately.

THE MAGIC OF PORRIDGE

Whole grains are a great food for anyone trying to maintain a healthy weight. The high fiber content of grains fills you up and slows digestion so that you stay fuller, longer. Grains also have a side benefit that makes them even more satisfying. When you cook a whole grain, you are rehydrating it with water.

According to the Volumetrics diet plan, foods that contain a lot of water, like fruits, vegetables, salads, and soups, provide the most satisfaction for the least amount of calories. When you eat a cup of soup, your body registers a feeling of fullness that is the same as if you ate a cup of cheese. It's all about volume, and finding foods that have a large, water-enhanced volume and are low in calories is the Volumetrics strategy.

So if you are looking to lose weight, consider porridge- and risotto-style cooking of your grains. For your pilaf, you probably want to cook brown rice with a 2-to-1 ratio of water to grain. But if you are really looking to maximize the feeling of fullness, consider cooking a risotto, with a 3- or 4-to-1 ratio. Or try the Savory Porridge on page 45, and simmer a blend of fiber-rich grains with a 4- or 5-to-1 ratio of water to grain.

All that water will expand your grains to a comforting, tender texture, and also make a small amount of grain into a huge, satisfying bowl of hearty food. Add some vegetables, and you only add to the effect.

That's a delicious way to keep the pounds off, all while enjoying your meals and no hunger pangs!

SAVORY PORRIDGE

Porridge *is a homely sounding name for an elemental food. Grains, cooked with enough water to break them into a thick, spoonable mixture, are probably one of the first foods people made from the harvest. The secret of these comforting hot breakfast bowls is that extra water makes them extra filling and helpful in aiding weight loss. Topped with some savory tidbits, they are a great start to the day.*

SERVES 4

1 cup mixed brown rice, spelt, barley, oats, or other grain

4 cups water

Pinch of salt

TOPPING SUGGESTIONS FOR 1 SERVING

2 eggs scrambled with 6 spears asparagus, 4 medium mushrooms, and 1 cup packed fresh spinach

4 ounces sliced, prebaked tofu, 1 cup steamed or raw broccoli, and ¼ cup kimchi

2 ounces smoked fish or turkey, 1 medium Roma tomato, chopped, ½ cup nonfat plain Greek yogurt, and Tabasco sauce to taste

½ cup drained black beans, ¼ cup salsa, ¼ cup thawed frozen corn, and ¼ cup nonfat plain Greek yogurt

Cook the porridge by combining the grains, water, and salt in either a 2-quart pot or a slow cooker. In a pot, bring to a boil, then lower to a simmer and cook for 1 hour. In a slow cooker, cook on high for 5 hours.

When the grains have burst and are thickening the porridge, stir well and transfer to a storage tub, or serve. For each serving, top 1¼ cups cooked porridge with the toppings of your choice.

Keeps for 1 week, tightly covered, in the refrigerator.

CINNAMON TOAST *and* FRUIT "CAPRESE"

Nobody needs to know that this colorful breakfast is actually a way to use up stale bread. An Italian nonna *would never let bread go to waste, so in the spirit of economy, try baking it with some cinnamon and sugar and tossing it with fruit and protein-rich fresh mozzarella.*

SERVES 4 TO 6

CROUTONS

4 cups cubed whole wheat bread

2 tablespoons unsalted butter, melted

2 teaspoons cinnamon

¼ cup packed light brown sugar

SALAD

4 medium ripe D'Anjou pears

2 cups fresh raspberries or other fruit

4 ounces fresh mozzarella, torn or sliced

2 tablespoons freshly squeezed lemon juice

1 tablespoon canola oil

Preheat the oven to 300°F. In a large bowl, drizzle the bread with the melted butter, then sprinkle with the cinnamon and brown sugar and toss to coat. Transfer to a rimmed baking sheet and bake for 40 minutes to 1 hour, stirring every 20 minutes, until the bread cubes are crisp. Let cool on a rack. Store the cooled croutons in an airtight container at room temperature.

For the salad, core and slice the pears into a large bowl. Add the raspberries and mozzarella. In a cup, stir together the lemon juice and oil and drizzle over the pear mixture. Add 2 cups of the cinnamon croutons and toss to combine. Let stand for 5 minutes or up to 1 hour to soften, and serve.

PUMPKIN PIE BAKED STEEL-CUT OATS

If you have ever enjoyed leftover pumpkin pie right out of the refrigerator, you under-stand just how wonderful this dish is. With all the familiar flavor of pumpkin pie (and pumpkin is a very healthy vegetable, you know), these oats will make a breakfast you will crave all year long.

SERVES 8

Butter, for the pan
1½ cups steel-cut oats
1 cup pumpkin purée
2 large eggs, whisked
½ cup maple syrup
1 teaspoon cinnamon
½ teaspoon ground cloves
¼ teaspoon ground nutmeg
½ teaspoon salt
1 cup milk
1½ cups warm water
1 teaspoon vanilla extract

Preheat the oven to 375°F. Butter a 2-quart casserole dish with a lid. In a small saucepan, toast the oats over medium-high heat, swirling the pan until they smell toasty. Take off the heat.

In a large bowl, mash the pumpkin purée and mix in the eggs, maple syrup, cinnamon, cloves, nutmeg, and salt. Whisk in the milk, water, and vanilla, then stir in the toasted oats.

Scrape into the prepared dish, smooth the top, and put the lid on. Bake for 50 to 55 minutes. If you shake the pan, it should jiggle but be set in the middle. Remove the lid and let cool for 10 minutes before serving.

Keeps for 1 week, tightly covered, in the refrigerator.

PEACHY YOGURT COFFEE CAKE

For times when only a coffee cake will do, bring this showstopper. The buttery streusel, tender and tangy peaches, and stealthy whole grain cake will wow everyone who tries a slice.

SERVES 10

STREUSEL

½ cup packed light brown sugar

¼ cup (½ stick) unsalted butter, melted

½ cup white whole wheat flour

¼ cup rolled oats

2 tablespoons cinnamon

¼ teaspoon salt

CAKE

1 cup white whole wheat flour

1 cup whole wheat pastry flour

2 teaspoons baking powder

½ teaspoon baking soda

½ teaspoon salt

1 cup buttermilk

1 teaspoon vanilla extract

½ cup (1 stick) unsalted butter, at room temperature, plus more for the pan

1 cup packed light brown sugar

2 large eggs, whisked

2 large peaches, chopped

Preheat the oven to 350°F. Butter a 10-inch round springform pan and wrap the bottom and outer sides of the pan with a piece of foil to prevent leaks.

In a medium bowl, combine the brown sugar, melted butter, white whole wheat flour, oats, cinnamon, and salt and stir to combine. Chill until the cake batter is ready.

For the cake, in a large bowl, combine the white whole wheat flour, pastry flour, baking powder, baking soda, and salt and whisk to combine.

In a medium bowl, whisk together the buttermilk and vanilla.

In a stand mixer fitted with the batter paddle, or in a large bowl using an electric mixer, beat the butter until fluffy. Scrape down and add the 1 cup brown sugar and beat until fluffy and light, about 4 minutes, scraping down to make sure it is evenly mixed. Beat in the eggs until the mixture is lightened in color, about 2 minutes.

With the mixer running on low, add one third of the flour mixture and mix to combine, then beat in half of the buttermilk mixture. Add another third of the flour mixture, beat until smooth, and scrape down. Beat in the remaining buttermilk mixture and, when combined, beat in the remaining flour mixture. Fold in the chopped peaches. Scrape the batter into the prepared pan and sprinkle with the streusel mixture. Bake for 50 to 55 minutes, or until a toothpick inserted into the center of the pan comes out with no wet batter clinging to it (there will be some peach juices, but no batter). Cool on a rack before serving.

Keeps for 1 week, tightly covered, at room temperature.

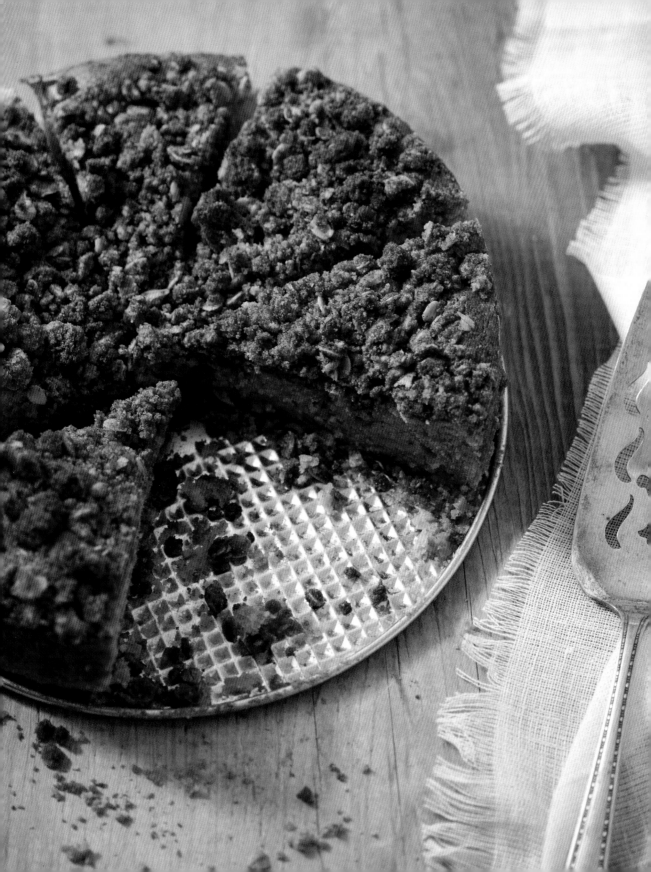

CINNAMON-APPLE BUTTER BARS

Apple butter is the magic ingredient in these bars, providing a thick, cinnamony filling so that you can put them together quickly. Pick a sweet cooking apple like Gala or Fuji, or a local favorite that isn't too tart.

SERVES 16

1 cup apple butter

1 large apple, peeled and chopped

Butter or canola oil, for the pan

2 cups rolled oats

1 cup whole wheat pastry flour

½ teaspoon salt

½ teaspoon baking powder

½ teaspoon baking soda

1 cup packed light brown sugar

½ cup milk

1 large egg, whisked

1 teaspoon vanilla extract

¼ cup (½ stick) unsalted butter, melted

Preheat the oven to 350°F. In a medium bowl, stir together the apple butter and chopped apple, and reserve. Grease a 9-inch square baking pan with 2-inch sides. In a large bowl, combine the oats, flour, salt, baking powder, baking soda, and brown sugar. Mix well. In a medium bowl, whisk together the milk, egg, and vanilla, then whisk in the melted butter.

Mix the milk mixture into the oat mixture and stir to combine. Spread a little more than half of the batter in the prepared pan and use wet hands to flatten it without sticking. Spread the apple mixture over the batter, then dollop the remaining batter over the filling. Bake for about 45 minutes, or until the edges are deep golden brown and the center of the bars wiggles only slightly when shaken. Let cool and cut 4 x 4 to make 16 bars.

Keeps for 1 week, tightly covered, in the refrigerator.

FRUITY CARROT MUFFINS

Bake up a batch of these muffins and you can enjoy them at home or on the go, with a schmear of cream cheese or even peanut butter. They are packed with sweet carrots and dried fruit, and the whole grains will keep you full until lunchtime.

SERVES 12

1 cup white whole wheat flour
1 cup whole wheat pastry flour
1 teaspoon cinnamon
1½ teaspoons baking soda
½ teaspoon salt
1 cup buttermilk
¼ cup canola oil, plus more for the pan
½ cup honey
1 large egg
1 cup dried apricots, chopped
1½ cups shredded carrot
¼ cup turbinado sugar

Preheat the oven to 350°F. Oil a 12-cup muffin pan or fill with paper liners. In a large bowl, mix together the flours, cinnamon, baking soda, and salt.

In another bowl, whisk together the buttermilk, canola oil, honey, and egg. Stir into the flour mixture. When almost mixed, stir in the apricots and carrot.

Scoop ¼-cup portions into the muffin cups, then sprinkle each with 1 teaspoon of turbinado sugar.

Bake for 30 minutes, or until a toothpick inserted in the center of a muffin comes out clean.

Cool for 10 minutes in the pan on a rack, then gently remove and cool completely.

YOGURT-COTTAGE CHEESE MUFFINS _with_ TARRAGON

Looking for a higher-protein muffin, with lots of great herby flavor? In this tangy, savory bread, yogurt and cottage cheese team up to produce a tender, moist muffin. The side effect of all that pale-colored yogurt is that the muffin looks like it's made with white flour, and nobody will care about anything but all that yummy cottage cheese.

SERVES 9

¼ cup canola oil, plus more for the pan
2 cups whole wheat pastry flour
1 teaspoon baking soda
½ teaspoon salt
1½ teaspoons dried tarragon
1 cup nonfat plain yogurt
1 large egg
¼ cup honey
1 cup low-fat cottage cheese

Preheat the oven to 375°F. Fill 9 muffin cups with paper liners, then spray or oil the top of the muffin pan.

In a large bowl, whisk together the flour, baking soda, salt, and tarragon. In a medium bowl, whisk together the yogurt, egg, honey, and oil. Quickly stir the yogurt mixture into the dry ingredients, then fold in the cottage cheese. Scoop the batter into the prepared muffin cups, filling them to the top.

Bake for 15 to 18 minutes, or until a toothpick inserted in the center of a muffin in the middle of the pan comes out clean. Cool completely in the pan on a rack.

Keeps for 1 week, tightly covered, in the refrigerator.

CHERRY *and* PINE NUT
BREAKFAST FOCACCIA

Adults and children alike love the idea of pizza for breakfast. This play on the pizza is topped with a sweet cherry sauce and dollops of creamy cheese, giving the lightly sweetened bread the look of a classic pizza pie. You have the option of tangy goat cheese, for more adult palates, or cream cheese, for a younger audience.

SERVES 4

¼ cup warm water

1 teaspoon active dry yeast

½ cup warm milk

¼ cup packed light brown sugar

¼ cup (½ stick) unsalted butter, melted, plus more for the pan

1 large egg

2 cups white whole wheat flour

½ teaspoon salt

1 (10-ounce) bag frozen dark cherries, thawed

2 teaspoons chopped fresh rosemary

2 tablespoons apple or other fruit juice, plus more as needed

1 tablespoon arrowroot

2 ounces cream cheese or soft goat cheese, crumbled

1 tablespoon pine nuts

2 tablespoons turbinado sugar

Butter a 12-inch circle on a sheet pan and reserve. Put the water in a cup, then stir in the yeast until dissolved. Put the yeast mixture in the bowl of a stand mixer or other bowl and let the mixture get foamy. Stir in the warm milk, brown sugar, butter, and egg, and then stir in the flour and salt. Make a soft dough and knead it for 5 minutes.

On the prepared sheet pan, flatten the dough to a 10- to 12-inch round. Cover and let rise for half an hour, until puffed.

Preheat the oven to 375°F.

While the dough rises, make the toppings. In a small saucepan, combine the cherries and rosemary and heat over medium until it starts to bubble. In a cup, stir together the fruit juice and arrowroot, then pour into the bubbling cherries, stirring constantly until the juices are clear and thick. Let cool to room temperature.

When the dough is puffed, top with the cooled cherries and the cream cheese, then sprinkle with the pine nuts and turbinado sugar. Bake for 15 to 20 minutes, or until golden. Cool on a rack. Serve warm or at room temperature.

Keeps for 4 days, tightly covered, in the refrigerator.

BREAKFAST PIZZA WITH STRAWBERRY SAUCE, RICOTTA, AND SWEET WALNUT "MEATBALLS"

Pat a whole grain polenta layer into a pan, top with strawberry sauce and nutty, sweet "meatballs," and you have a fun alternative to a bowl of hot cereal, built to please the eye. These sweet "meatballs" are crave-worthy—you may want to make them on their own to garnish your hot cereal.

SERVES 8

Canola oil, for the pan

1 cup millet, steel-cut oats, or buckwheat groats

2½ cups water

Pinch of salt

2 tablespoons packed light brown sugar or honey

1 cup ricotta cheese

2 cups frozen strawberries, thawed

¼ cup granulated sugar

2 tablespoons apple juice

2 teaspoons arrowroot or cornstarch

"MEATBALLS"

½ cup walnuts

¼ cup packed pitted dates

¼ cup rolled oats

Pinch of salt

2 tablespoons apple juice

Oil a 10-inch round springform pan. In a 1-quart pot, dry-toast the grain by swirling the pan over medium-high heat. Add the water and bring to a boil. Cover tightly and cook for about 25 minutes, or until all the water is absorbed. Take off the heat and stir. The grains will break up to make it sticky. Stir in the salt and the brown sugar. Spread the grain in the prepared pan and smooth with the back of a wet spoon. Let cool.

Preheat the oven to 400°F.

Scoop the ricotta cheese onto a double layer of paper towels to drain any extra water.

In a 1-quart pot, combine the strawberries and granulated sugar and place over medium heat. Bring to a bubble, until the juices are flowing from the fruit. In a cup, whisk together the apple juice and arrowroot, then stir into the fruit. The mixture will boil and thicken very quickly. Take off the heat, then spread the strawberry sauce on the grain crust.

For the "meatballs," in a food processor, pulse the walnuts, dates, oats, and salt to make a coarse purée.
Add the apple juice and process to a paste.

Dollop heaping tablespoons of ricotta over the strawberry sauce, then scoop tablespoon-sized portions of the walnut mixture, form into balls, and arrange over the pie.

Bake for 25 to 30 minutes, or until the walnut balls are firm to the touch. Let cool for 5 minutes before slicing and serving.

Keeps for 4 days, tightly covered, in the refrigerator.

BISCUIT-TOPPED BREAKFAST PIE

Biscuits and gravy is an ever-popular diner staple, and this easy recipe puts it in a pie. Throw in some veggies and lightened-up gravy, and it's actually much better for you than the original. Vegetarians can use their favorite meatless sausage, too.

SERVES 6 TO 9

2 teaspoons canola oil, plus more for the pan

1 large onion, chopped

2 large carrots, chopped

3 (4-ounce) cooked chicken sausages (apple, sage, or plain), sliced

¼ cup white whole wheat flour

1 cup milk

1 cup chicken or vegetable stock

2 teaspoons dried sage

1 teaspoon dried thyme

2 cups (2 ounces) fresh baby spinach, chopped

½ teaspoon salt

½ teaspoon freshly ground black pepper

2 cups homemade baking mix (page 61)

¾ cup plain yogurt

Flour, for shaping

Preheat the oven to 400°F. Lightly oil a 9-inch square baking pan. In a 4-quart pot, heat the canola oil over medium-high heat and sauté the onion, carrots, and sausage until the onion is golden and the carrots are softened, about 5 minutes. Sprinkle the white whole wheat flour over the vegetables in the pan and stir to coat the veggies and sausage, scraping the bottom of the pan as you stir. Continue stirring for a couple of minutes to brown the flour a little. Take the pan off the heat and stir in the milk gradually, stirring to incorporate the flour before adding the rest of the milk and then the stock. Stir in the sage and thyme, return the pan to the heat, and simmer until the sauce thickens, about 3 minutes. Stir in the spinach and salt and pepper, then take off the heat and stir to wilt the spinach. Transfer to the prepared baking pan.

In a large bowl, combine the biscuit mix and yogurt and mix together, kneading gently to incorporate the flour. On a floured counter, pat out the dough into an 8-inch square. Cut 3 x 3 to make 9 squares, then place the biscuits over the sausage mixture in the baking pan.

Bake for 20 to 25 minutes, or until the biscuits are deep golden brown and the sauce is bubbling around the sides. Serve warm.

Once cooled, keeps for 4 days, tightly covered, in the refrigerator.

PUFFY BAKED APPLE PANCAKE

This big, showy cake is not any harder to make than a batch of regular pancakes, but somehow it gets relegated to "for company only" status. Sauté some apples, or branch out with other fruit, and complement them with this puffy, eggy cake for a crowd-pleasing breakfast treat!

SERVES 4

APPLES

¼ cup (½ stick) unsalted butter, divided

2 cups peeled and chopped apples

2 tablespoons packed light brown sugar

1 tablespoon freshly squeezed lemon juice

BATTER

3 large eggs

¾ cup milk

½ cup white whole wheat flour

2 tablespoons granulated sugar

Pinch of ground nutmeg

¼ teaspoon salt

2 tablespoons confectioners' sugar (optional)

Preheat the oven to 425°F. Melt a tablespoon of the butter in a 9-inch round cake pan and swirl to coat. In a large sauté pan, melt the remaining butter and sauté the apples over medium-high heat. When the apples are soft and golden, add the brown sugar and lemon juice and cook until almost dry. Take off the heat and scrape into a large bowl to cool.

For the batter, in a blender, combine the eggs and milk and blend on high for 1 minute, then add the flour, granulated sugar, nutmeg, and salt. Blend on high until well mixed and frothy. Pour the batter over the apples in the bowl and stir to mix, then pour into the prepared cake pan. Bake for 14 to 15 minutes, or until puffed and golden.

Sift confectioners' sugar over the cake, if desired, and serve in wedges while hot.

BIG CINNAMON-OAT PANCAKES *with* BERRIES

Studded with berries and chewy flecks of oat, these jumbo cakes will satisfy a hungry breakfast lover. Pancakes are pure comfort and pleasure, and they hardly take any effort at all. Your family will be so happy to get pancakes that they will never wonder whether they are made with healthy whole grain flours.

SERVES 6 TO 8

1½ cups whole wheat pastry flour

¼ cup rolled oats

1 tablespoon packed light brown sugar

½ teaspoon cinnamon

1 teaspoon baking powder

¼ teaspoon baking soda

¼ teaspoon salt

1½ cups buttermilk

2 tablespoons canola oil

½ teaspoon vanilla extract

Canola oil, for the pan

1 cup fresh blueberries or raspberries

Grade B maple syrup, for serving

In a large bowl, combine the flour, oats, brown sugar, cinnamon, baking powder, baking soda, and salt. In a medium bowl, whisk together the buttermilk, canola oil, and vanilla and quickly stir into the dry mixture.

Put a large griddle or nonstick pan over medium heat. When hot, brush lightly with oil. Scoop level ⅓-cup portions of batter onto the hot pan, leaving room for the cakes to spread. Use the back of the cup to spread into 6-inch rounds. Drop 2 tablespoons of berries onto each cake and tap them down into the batter. Cook for a minute, then reduce the heat to medium-low. Cook until the edges look done and the batter is bubbly, about 4 minutes. (Every pan and stove is different; it may take more or less time.) Carefully flip the pancakes and cook for another 3 to 4 minutes on that side. Serve hot with maple syrup.

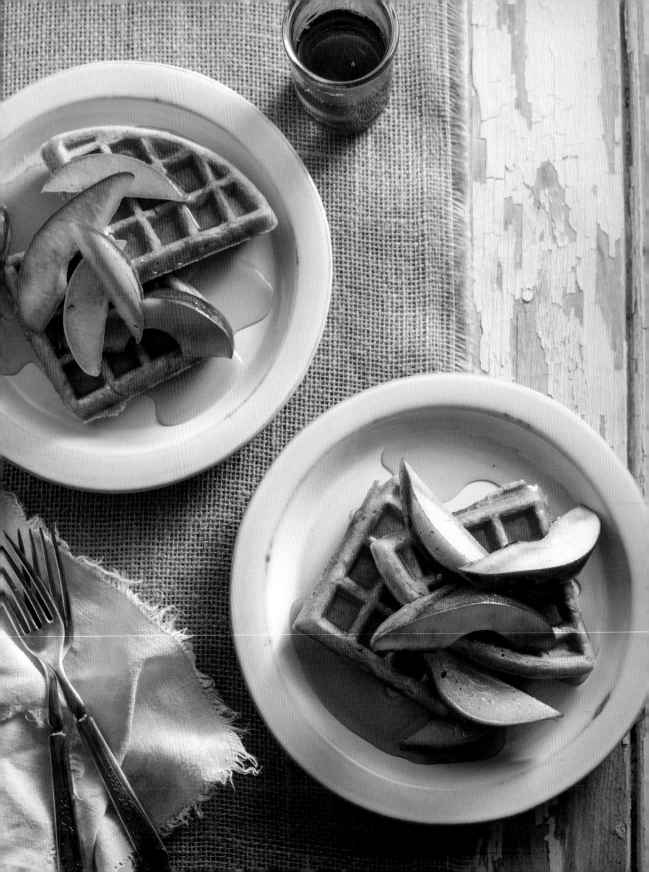

OVERNIGHT WHOLE WHEAT WAFFLES
ᴡɪᴛʜ MAPLE-PEAR SAUCE

Once you buy a waffle iron, you need a great whole grain waffle recipe to do it justice. These fluffy, crisp waffles rely on an overnight rise with yeast and a quick mix with eggs and baking soda in the morning. The slow ferment gives them character and depth of flavor. Perfect for soaking up a fruity burst of pure maple and pears.

SERVES 5

2 cups milk

¼ cup canola oil

2 tablespoons granulated sugar

½ teaspoon salt

½ cup warm water

2 teaspoons active dry yeast

3 cups whole wheat pastry flour

½ cup white whole wheat or
  unbleached white flour

2 teaspoons cinnamon

2 large eggs

¼ teaspoon baking soda

Melted butter for waffle iron

SAUCE

5 large ripe pears

¾ cup maple syrup

½ teaspoon vanilla extract

In a small pot over medium heat, combine the milk and canola oil and heat until hot to the touch. Stir in the sugar and salt, then remove from the heat and let cool to lukewarm.

In a large bowl, combine the water and yeast. Let stand until foamy, about 5 minutes.

Add the warm milk mixture to the yeast and stir. Whisk in the flours and cinnamon. Cover and let stand (or refrigerate) until doubled in volume, 2 to 3 hours at room temperature or overnight in the refrigerator. In the morning, take the batter out and let stand in a warm place for half an hour to warm up.

Heat a waffle iron and preheat the oven to 200°F (to hold the finished waffles). Whisk together the eggs and baking soda, then fold into the waffle batter. Using a pastry brush or paper towel, lightly coat the waffle iron with melted butter. Cook the waffles (using about ½ cup batter per waffle) until golden and crisp. Butter the iron in between batches as needed. Serve the waffles immediately as they are ready, or keep them warm in the oven until ready to serve.

For the sauce, chop the pears (peel them first, if desired) and put them in a 4-quart pot with the maple syrup and vanilla. Bring to a boil, then remove from the heat. (Don't boil for long, or the juices of the pears will thin the syrup.) Serve warm over the waffles. Makes 2½ cups sauce.

BREADS

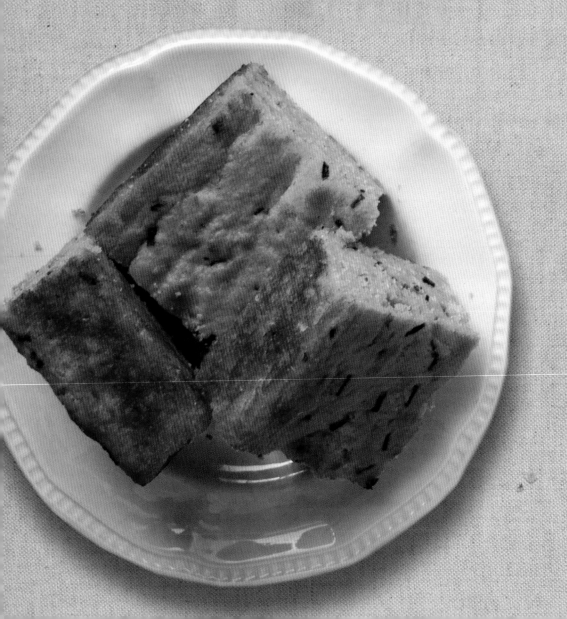

MAKE YOUR OWN BAKING MIX

For everyone who has ever said, "I don't have time to bake," I created this recipe. Simply stir up this mix and keep it in jars in the fridge, and you will be several steps closer to hot, toasty, homemade biscuits, scones, and pancakes. All natural and economical, too.

MAKES 4 CUPS

1½ cups whole wheat pastry flour

2 cups white whole wheat flour
  (can substitute 1 cup with unbleached flour)

2 teaspoons baking powder

2 teaspoons baking soda

½ teaspoon salt

2 tablespoons granulated sugar

¼ cup (½ stick) unsalted butter, chilled

In a large bowl, combine the flours, baking powder, baking soda, salt, and sugar. Whisk until evenly combined. Using a box grater, shred the butter on the coarse holes into the flour, tossing to coat. Mix with your hands, squeezing to coat some of the butter with flour, but leaving the butter in small pieces. At this point, store the mix in airtight jars or resealable plastic bags in the refrigerator or freezer.

BAKING-MIX BISCUITS

In the time that it takes to preheat the oven, you can have biscuits mixed, shaped, and on the pan. Hot biscuits make a simple soup or salad into an exciting meal. You can always add a sprinkling of your favorite herb, spice, or shredded cheese to complement the main course.

SERVES 8

2 cups homemade baking mix
³/₄ cup nonfat plain yogurt
Flour, for shaping

Preheat the oven to 400°F and line a sheet pan with parchment paper or lightly oil it. Measure the mix into a large bowl and stir in the yogurt. The dough will be stiff. Gather and squeeze the dough gently just to incorporate all the flour. Don't overmix or it will make tough biscuits.

In the bowl or on a floured counter, pat the dough into a ³/₄-inch-thick rectangle or disk. Cut into 8 squares or wedges and transfer to the baking sheet.

Bake for 12 minutes, or until golden brown. Transfer to a rack to cool.

BAKING-MIX PANCAKES

SERVES 6

2 cups homemade baking mix
1 large egg
1¹/₂ cups buttermilk
Canola oil, for the pan

Measure the baking mix into a large bowl. In a cup, whisk the egg with the buttermilk, then stir into the mix.

Preheat a griddle or large skillet over medium-high heat. When hot, oil lightly (use a paper towel or pastry brush) and scoop ¹/₄-cup portions of batter onto the hot pan. Cook until the surface is covered with bubbles and the edges look dry, then flip. Cook for another minute or so, then transfer to a plate and serve.

BAKING-MIX SCONES

Your coffeehouse favorite is even better when baked at home and studded with your choice of fruits, nuts, or even chocolate chips. Dried fruit works best, but you can use fresh blueberries or raspberries if you fold them in very carefully at the end to keep them intact.

SERVES 8

2 cups homemade baking mix

¼ cup granulated sugar

¼ cup nonfat plain yogurt

2 large eggs

½ teaspoon vanilla extract (optional)

½ cup chopped dried fruit, chopped nuts, or chocolate chips

Flour, for shaping

1 large egg whisked with 1 tablespoon water, for glazing (optional)

Turbinado sugar, for topping (optional)

Preheat the oven to 400°F and line a sheet pan with parchment paper or lightly oil it. In a large bowl, combine the baking mix with the granulated sugar. In a medium bowl, whisk the yogurt with the eggs, then whisk in the vanilla, if desired. Quickly stir until nearly mixed, then stir in the dried fruit, nuts, or chocolate chips.

On a floured counter, form a disk of dough about an inch thick, then cut into 8 wedges. Transfer to the prepared baking sheet. If desired, brush the tops of the scones with egg wash and/or sprinkle them with turbinado sugar.

Bake for 13 to 15 minutes. Cool on a rack.

NO-KNEAD "STEALTH" BREAD

This recipe uses the stealth technique to gradually introduce whole grains— you can choose the level of whole wheat each time you bake. Why make no-knead bread? Because while the dough rests in the refrigerator, yeasts are slowly fermenting the flours, making the resulting bread more digestible, flavorful, and open textured. If you want the loaf to rise a little higher, you can replace 2 tablespoons of the flour with gluten flour for a little more structure.

SERVES 10

2½ teaspoons active dry yeast

1 tablespoon light brown sugar

2¼ cups warm water (105°F to 115°F) for 100% whole wheat bread, 2 cups for 75%, and 1¾ cups for 50%

1¼ teaspoons salt

4¼ cups white whole wheat flour for 100% whole wheat bread, 3½ cups white whole wheat flour and 1 cup unbleached flour for 75%, and 2¼ cups white whole wheat flour and 2¼ cups unbleached flour for 50%

3 tablespoons canola oil

Shortening, for the pan

In a large liquid measuring cup, stir the yeast and brown sugar into the water and let stand for about 20 minutes, or until it starts to bubble. In a square or rectangular storage tub with a lid (preferably 9 inches wide to line up with your baking pan), measure the salt and flours and stir. When the yeast has bloomed, stir the canola oil into the water and yeast mixture, then stir that into the flour mixture. Stir just until mixed. It will be loose, lumpy, and sticky. Cover with a damp towel or loosely with the lid of the tub. Let stand for 20 minutes, to relax the dough. Then, use a spatula to fold a third of the dough toward the center, then gently flip the other third of the dough over that and with wet hands, gently flatten. Let stand for 10 minutes, then rotate the dough to approach it from a different side and repeat the folding process. Do this again in 10 minutes, for a total of three folds. Then let the dough sit, loosely covered, for 2 hours, or until the batter rises to double the volume. Cover and refrigerate overnight, or for up to 2 days.

To bake, take the dough out of the refrigerator and let warm on the counter for a few minutes. If it is cooler than 75°F in your kitchen, turn your oven to 250°F for 5 minutes (then turn it off), so you can put the cold dough in a warm oven to help it rise. Heavily grease an 8½ x 4½-inch metal loaf pan with shortening. Using a rubber spatula, roll the dough gently over itself, forming a cylinder, and gently pinch to seal the seam. Trying not to deflate the dough, roll it out into the loaf pan, seam-side down. If the top of the dough looks torn or shaggy, wet your fingers and smooth it gently. It will not change much during its rise and baking, so make it pretty. Cover loosely with a damp kitchen towel or plastic wrap. Let stand for 2 hours, in or on top of the warm oven or in another warm spot, until the dough has risen to ½ inch or more above the rim of the pan.

Preheat the oven to 375°F. Bake the loaf for 35 minutes, or until the loaf sounds hollow when tapped with a finger. Cool on a rack for 10 minutes before gently tapping the loaf out onto the rack to finish cooling. Cool completely before slicing or storing. Keeps for one week wrapped in a paper towel in a plastic bag.

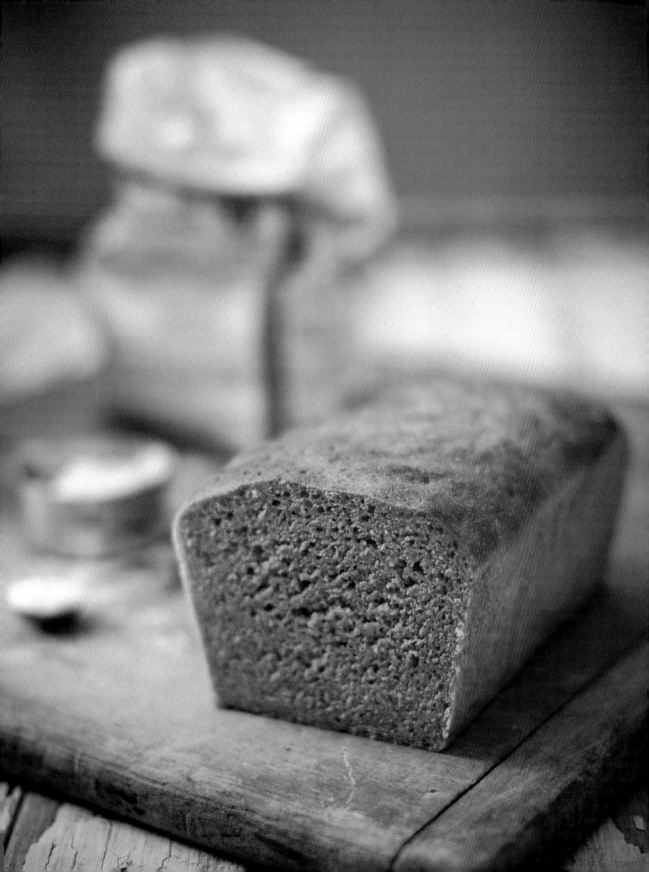

WHY OVERNIGHT? WHY FOLD?

No-knead, overnight, and refrigerated bread dough recipes have grown in popularity in recent years for several reasons. A big part of it is that we now understand more about how gluten forms structure in dough and that a slow rise in the refrigerator actually allows the dough to form gluten without kneading. This is especially helpful with whole wheat flour breads, because the bits of bran and germ in the dough can act like little knives, if you can imagine that, chopping the gluten into pieces during the kneading process. Whole wheat flour will always be a little lower in gluten than white flour, just because bran and germ take up volume but contribute no gluten. This lower gluten content, combined with the chopping action and weight of bran and germ, can make your whole grain bread dense and chewy.

Thanks to some thoughtful bakers and food chemists, we now know that treating the bread dough more gently will nurture the gluten that we need for structure. That's where folding comes in. White whole wheat flour, used throughout this book, has a more fragile form of gluten. It benefits from being gently stretched and folded, just a bit, instead of kneading. The bonus is that letting the yeast start work in the refrigerator also breaks down some of the indigestible parts of the wheat and adds more complexity to the flavor of the finished bread.

The bonus for you is that you don't have to knead! Just be patient, since you are asking a colony of microscopic yeasts to lift a pretty heavy load. When you take your refrigerated dough out, give it time to warm up and rise fully before baking.

SWITCHING WHOLE WHEAT FLOUR FOR WHITE: HYDRATION MATTERS

You may have tried baking a favorite bread or muffin with whole wheat flour instead of white, simply by substituting an equal measure of whole wheat for white. If your results were dry, heavy, and disappointing, you may just have needed one little tip. Whole grain flours absorb more liquids than white flours, so you need to adjust the ratio of water to flour for a good result. Bakers call the ratio of water to flour a measure of "hydration" and recommend making whole grain breads with a ratio of 70 to 75% water to 25 to 30% flour, measured by weight, not volume. Lack of awareness of this one bit of chemistry may be to blame for millions of loaves of heavy, unappealing bread! In the "stealth" bread and pizza crust recipes, you will see that adjustments have been made to allow a gradual increase in white whole wheat flour, with a higher ratio of water to flour (by weight, not volume).

OVERNIGHT "STEALTH" PIZZA DOUGH

Pizza is one of the most beloved foods in America and often criticized for its junk-food status. There's no reason that a pizza can't be made with stealthy addition of whole grain flour and topped with vegetables and lean proteins, making it the opposite of junk! Just have some restraint: spread your sauce thinly and keep the toppings light, or your pizza will be overloaded and soggy. The dough is best if you use it within three to four days; if you store it for a week, it gets a little more tangy but still works.

SERVES 4

2 cups white whole wheat flour for 100% whole wheat crust, 1³⁄₄ cups white whole wheat flour and ¹⁄₂ cup unbleached flour for 75%, and 1 cup white whole wheat flour and 1¹⁄₄ cups unbleached flour for 50%

³⁄₄ teaspoon salt

2 teaspoons active dry yeast

1 cup water

1 tablespoon extra-virgin olive oil, plus more for the tub

Flour, for shaping

Cornmeal, for the pan

In a large bowl, combine the flour, salt, and yeast, and stir to mix. In a liquid measuring cup, stir together the water and olive oil and then stir that into the flour. It will become stiff; you can switch to mixing with your hands, if needed. It will also be somewhat sticky. Let the dough rest for a few minutes, then divide into two even portions. Form two rounds of dough by tucking the edges of each piece of dough into the middle and working your way around until a circle is formed.

Lightly oil a storage tub and place the dough rounds in it, cover tightly, and chill overnight.

An hour or two before you are ready to make pizza, take out the dough that you plan to use (you can keep one of the portions refrigerated and use it later) and place on a lightly floured counter. Press and flatten the dough, flipping it to coat with flour. The warmth of your hands will help warm the dough. Cover the dough to prevent it from drying out as you let it come to room temperature and start to rise for at least an hour. Prepare the toppings for your pizza and reserve.

When the dough is warm and puffed, preheat the oven to 425°F.

Press and stretch the dough to a 12-inch round for a thin pizza, or larger for a cracker crust. Place on a cornmeal-dusted pan or pizza peel and top lightly with sauce and toppings. Bake on the bottom shelf of the oven for 15 minutes, or until the crust is golden brown and firm when you lift an edge with your spatula.

Transfer the hot pizza to a cutting board, cut into wedges or squares, and serve.

SOFT BUTTERMILK BUNS

Craving a pillowy roll to serve with your holiday feast or alongside a bowl of soup? Buttermilk has a wonderful tanginess that also tenderizes anything it is mixed with. Whole grain flours meld with the creamy buttermilk for a winner of a bun.

SERVES 14

½ cup warm water (105°F to 115°F)
4 tablespoons packed light brown sugar, divided
2 teaspoons active dry yeast
¾ cup buttermilk
1 cup rolled oats
6 tablespoons unsalted butter, melted
1 teaspoon salt
1 large egg
2½ cups white whole wheat flour
Canola oil, for the bowl and pans

In the bowl of a stand mixer or a large bowl, combine the water, 2 tablespoons of brown sugar, and the yeast and stir. Let the yeast bloom until bubbly, about 5 minutes.

With the dough hook or a wooden spoon, mix in the buttermilk, oats, butter, salt, and egg. Mix in the flour to make a soft dough. Knead for about 5 minutes.

Oil a large bowl and transfer the dough to the bowl. Coat the dough ball with oil by turning it over, then cover the bowl with plastic wrap or a damp kitchen towel. Let the dough rise until doubled, about an hour.

Preheat the oven to 375°F and lightly oil two large sheet pans.

Tear off balls of dough about the size of small apricots, or the size that you desire—they will end up twice that size after baking.

Form the balls and place on the oiled pans with 3 inches of space between them. Let rise for at least 45 minutes or 1 hour, or until doubled in size.

Bake for 15 to 20 minutes, or until the buns are golden brown and puffed. Roll one over and tap it with your finger; it should sound hollow.

Transfer to racks to cool. These keep in an airtight storage container for up to 1 week.

SAVORY GRANOLA CROUTONS FOR SALAD OR SOUP

Savory granolas are a growing phenomenon. I first had one on a composed salad in an upscale restaurant in San Francisco. Of course, your savory granola "croutons" may be floated on a soup, used to garnish a pasta or pizza, eaten with plain yogurt, or simply eaten out of hand. I take a stash of them to work with me for a non-sweet, energizing snack.

SERVES 12 (MAKES ABOUT 6 CUPS)

2 cups rolled oats

½ cup buckwheat groats

½ cup oat flour (grind ½ cup rolled oats in the blender to make flour)

¼ cup raw sunflower or hemp seeds

¼ cup sesame seeds

½ cup walnuts, chopped

1 teaspoon salt

½ teaspoon paprika

½ teaspoon dried thyme

½ teaspoon dried oregano

2 large egg whites, or 2 tablespoons ground flax seeds

¼ cup extra-virgin olive oil, plus more for the pan

¼ cup apple juice

¼ cup shredded Parmesan cheese (optional)

Preheat the oven to 350°F. Lightly oil a large rimmed sheet pan and set aside.

In a large bowl, combine the oats, buckwheat, oat flour, sunflower seeds, sesame seeds, walnuts, salt, paprika, thyme, and oregano and mix well. In a medium bowl, whisk the egg whites, or if using flax seeds, whisk the flax with ¼ cup water and let stand for 5 minutes to thicken. Add the olive oil and apple juice and whisk to blend. Stir into the oat mixture and if using Parmesan, stir that in at the same time.

Spread the oat mixture over the oiled pan evenly and press into a flat layer with the back of a large spoon.

Bake for 20 minutes, then use a large metal spatula to gently turn large sections of the mixture, trying not to break it up. Bake for 10 minutes longer, then cool in the pan on a rack.

Transfer to an airtight storage container. Keeps for 2 weeks at room temperature.

BASIC CROUTONS _with_ VARIATIONS

Once you have invested in a hearty, whole grain loaf, the last thing you want is for it to go to waste. Enter the crouton, an easy method of using up your bread, all while adding whole grains to salads and soups. Croutons keep well, too. Store them for up to a month once they are crisp and dry.

SERVES 8 (MAKES 4 CUPS)

4 cups cubed whole wheat bread (size of cubes is up to you)
3 tablespoons olive oil or unsalted butter, plus more for the pans
1 teaspoon dried herbs or spices (pick a blend or a single herb)
2 garlic cloves, crushed
½ teaspoon fine salt
¼ cup finely grated hard cheese, such as Parmesan or manchego (optional)

Preheat the oven to 300°F. Lightly oil two rimmed baking sheets. Put the bread cubes in a large bowl. In a microwave-safe ramekin or in a small sauté pan, heat the oil or butter just to warm, then add the herbs, garlic, and salt. Stir just until fragrant, then pour over the bread cubes. Scrape the seasonings from the ramekin or pan and stir in. Toss the bread cubes to coat.

Spread the bread cubes on the sheet pans and bake for 20 minutes, then stir. Bake for 20 minutes more if the cubes are small. If the cubes are larger, add more time.

To add cheese, 10 minutes before you anticipate the croutons will be done, sprinkle the cheese over the hot croutons in the pan and return to the oven for the remaining 10 minutes.

Cool on racks before transferring to airtight jars or containers.

Keeps for a couple of weeks, tightly covered, at room temperature.

SAVORY SPINACH QUICK BREAD

As long as you are eating bread, you might as well have a bit of vegetable, too.
This quick and easy loaf is swirled with deep green spinach, so you have a head
start on your veggie servings before you even start piling them on the sandwich.

SERVES 10

4 cups (4 ounces) fresh baby spinach

2 teaspoons dried thyme

3 large eggs

½ cup honey

½ cup canola oil, plus more for the pan

½ cup milk

2 cups white whole wheat flour

1 cup unbleached flour

2 teaspoons baking powder

1 teaspoon baking soda

1 teaspoon salt

Preheat the oven to 350°F. Lightly oil a 9 x 5-inch loaf pan.

In a food processor, mince the spinach with the dried thyme. Add the eggs, honey, canola oil, and milk and pulse until combined. (Hold a folded kitchen towel over the feed tube as you pulse the food processor so that the liquids won't spatter.)

In a large bowl, whisk together the flours, baking powder, baking soda, and salt. Scrape the spinach mixture into the flour mixture and stir just until combined.

Transfer the batter to the prepared pan and smooth the top. Bake for 50 to 55 minutes, or until the top is golden brown and cracked a little and a toothpick inserted into the center comes out with no wet batter clinging to it.

Cool in the pan on a rack. When completely cool, wrap tightly or store in a resealable plastic bag. Keeps for 1 week in the refrigerator.

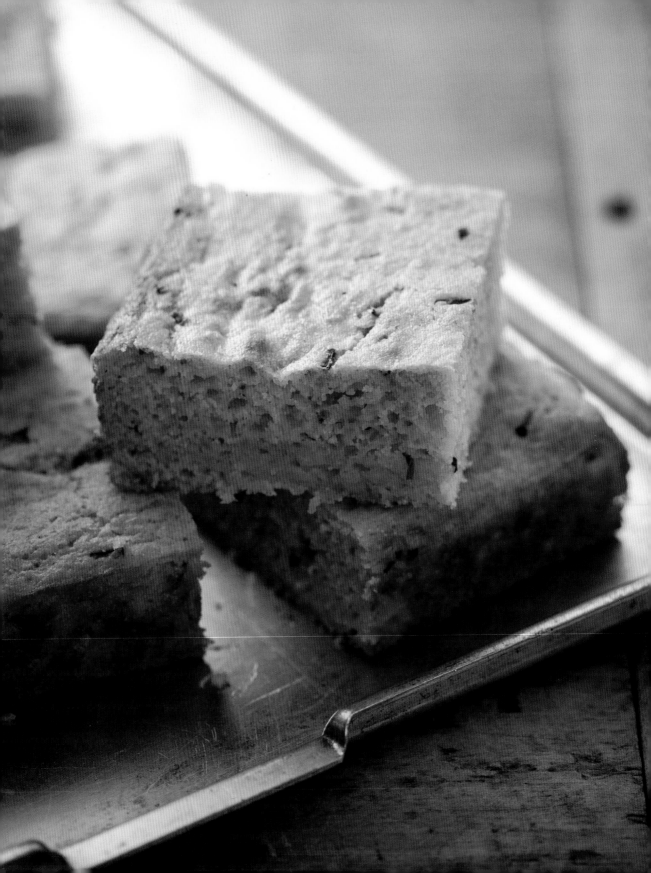

CHEDDAR-CHIVE CORNBREAD

Cornbread is iconic, especially down South, where every home cook has a jazzed-up recipe of her own. This moist, delectable version is laced with savory Cheddar cheese and zingy chives. Make sure to use whole grain cornmeal, not the de-germinated kind, for all the corn flavor you crave.

SERVES 9

1¼ cups yellow cornmeal

¾ cup white whole wheat flour

¼ cup packed light brown sugar

2 teaspoons baking powder

1 teaspoon baking soda

1 teaspoon salt

1 large egg

1¾ cups buttermilk

¼ cup canola oil, plus more for the pan

¼ cup minced chives

8 ounces sharp Cheddar cheese, shredded (1½ cups)

Preheat the oven to 400°F and oil or butter a 9-inch square baking pan, preferably metal. In a large bowl, whisk together the cornmeal, flour, brown sugar, baking powder, baking soda, and salt. In a medium bowl, whisk the egg, then whisk in the buttermilk and canola oil.

Quickly stir the buttermilk mixture into the cornmeal mixture. Stir in the chives and cheese just to combine, then scrape the batter into the prepared pan. Smooth the top and bake for 20 to 25 minutes, or until the top is golden brown and a toothpick inserted in the center of the bread comes out dry.

Serve warm, or cool completely before wrapping tightly and storing in the refrigerator for up to 1 week.

CHERRY-ALMOND QUICK BREAD

This tender bread, studded with sweet-tart cherries and laced with almond flavor, will wow anyone who tries it. A dusting of crunchy almonds and sugar on top gives it plenty of curb appeal.

SERVES 8

2½ cups white whole wheat flour
¾ cup packed light brown sugar
1 teaspoon baking powder
1 teaspoon baking soda
½ teaspoon salt
3 large eggs
1 cup buttermilk
½ cup canola oil, plus more for the pan
2 teaspoons almond extract
1 cup dried cherries
3 tablespoons turbinado sugar
¼ cup slivered almonds, finely chopped

Preheat the oven to 350°F. Oil a 9½ x 5½-inch metal loaf pan.

In a large bowl, combine the flour, brown sugar, baking powder, baking soda, and salt. In a medium bowl, whisk the eggs, then whisk in the buttermilk, oil, and almond extract. Stir the egg mixture into the flour mixture and when combined, stir in the cherries. Scrape into the loaf pan and smooth the top. Sprinkle with the turbinado sugar and almonds.

Bake for 45 to 55 minutes, or until golden brown and a toothpick inserted in the center of the loaf comes out dry.

Cool the loaf in the pan on a rack for about 10 minutes. Gently remove the loaf and let it cool until it reaches room temperature, then wrap tightly or place in an airtight storage bag. Keeps for 1 week in the refrigerator or at room temperature.

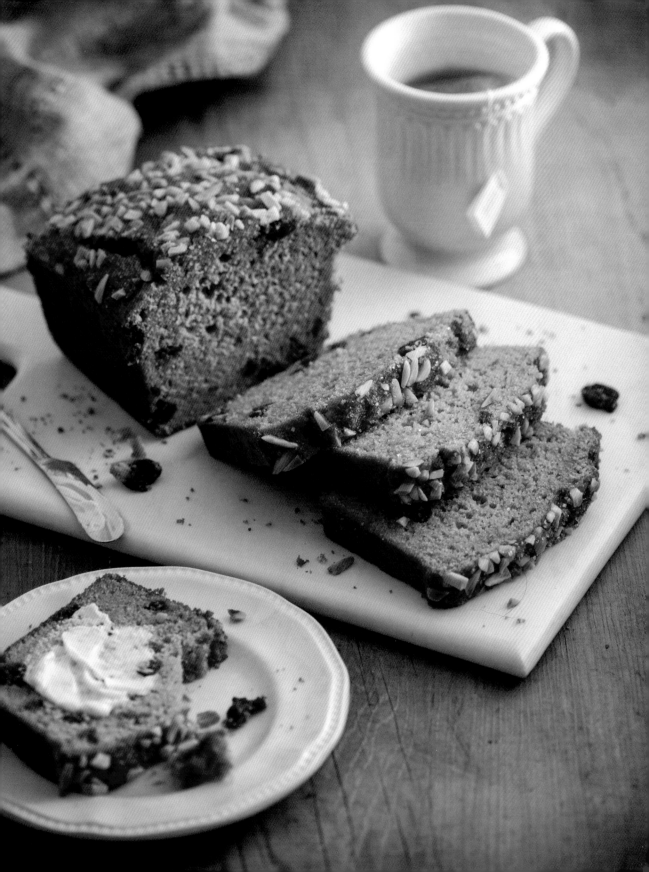

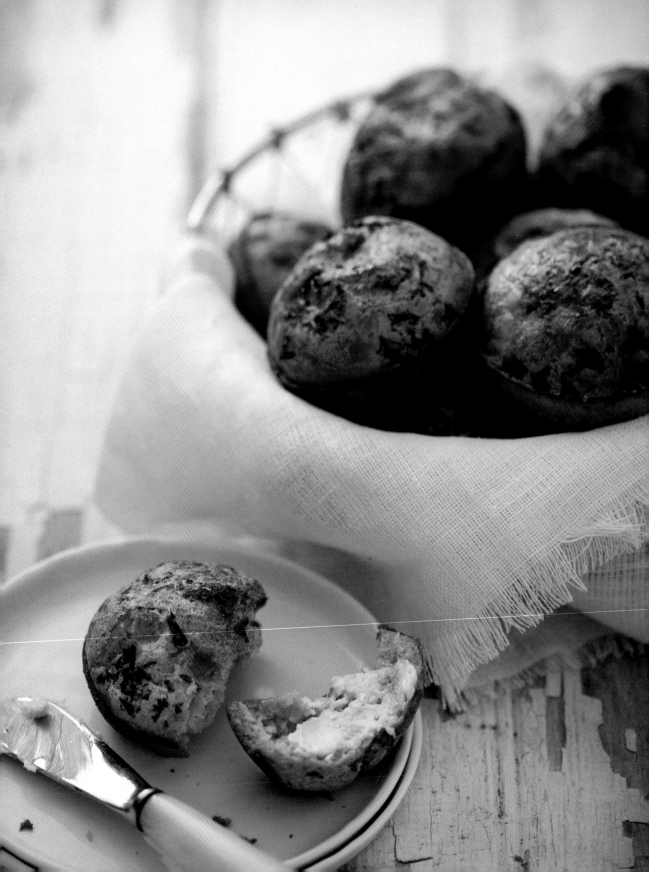

PARSLEY-PARMESAN POPOVERS

Popovers make any dinner extra special—even canned soup is a fabulous meal when you have piping-hot, golden popovers for dipping. These come out beautifully when baked in a standard muffin tin, but if you have a special popover pan, they will be a little taller.

SERVES 8

Butter, for the pan

1 cup whole milk

1 tablespoon canola or extra-virgin olive oil

2 large eggs

1 cup whole wheat pastry flour

$\frac{1}{2}$ teaspoon salt

$\frac{1}{8}$ cup minced fresh parsley

$\frac{1}{4}$ cup shredded Parmesan cheese

Thoroughly grease 8 cups of a muffin tin or popover pan.

Whisk the milk, oil, and eggs together until well combined. Add the flour and salt and blend until there are no lumps.

Combine the parsley and Parmesan in a small bowl.

Use a $\frac{1}{3}$-cup measure to fill the muffin tins three quarters full of batter. Sprinkle a couple teaspoons of the parsley-Parmesan mixture over each popover.

Place in a cold oven and set it to 450°F. Bake for 25 minutes, or until the popovers are puffed and light brown. Reduce the heat to 350°F. Bake for another 15 minutes so that the popovers are crisp and firm.

Serve warm.

SALADS

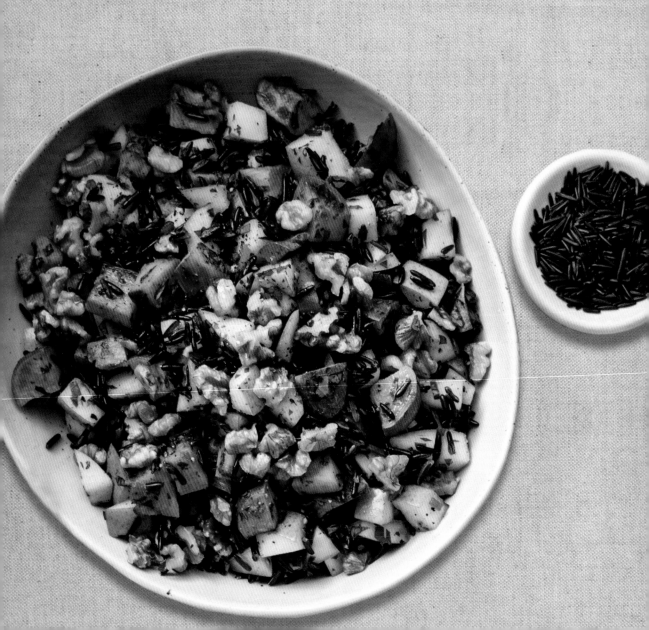

KALE *and* TOMATO CAESAR SALAD

Kale salads are here to stay—especially this one, crowned with hearty whole grain croutons. If you haven't learned to love anchovies, you can leave them out, although chances are that when you have enjoyed a Caesar salad in a restaurant, there was anchovy paste in the dressing.

SERVES 4

1 cup Basic Croutons (page 70) or Savory
  Granola Croutons (page 69)

2 ounces shredded Parmesan cheese, divided

1 garlic clove, peeled

1 teaspoon Dijon mustard

½ teaspoon Worcestershire sauce

1 tablespoon anchovy paste (optional)

3 tablespoons freshly squeezed lemon juice

¼ cup extra-virgin olive oil

1 bunch (8 ounces) stemmed kale or romaine lettuce, chopped

2 large heirloom or beefsteak tomatoes, cut into wedges

Prepare the croutons and let cool.

In a food processor, place half of the Parmesan cheese and the garlic clove and process to a smooth purée. Add the Dijon, Worcestershire, anchovy paste (if using), and lemon juice and process until smooth. Gradually add the olive oil with the machine running. Transfer the dressing to a small bowl.

For tender kale, place it in a large bowl, add dressing, and massage it a bit by scrunching it in your hands to tenderize the leaves.

In a large salad bowl, toss together the kale, tomatoes, croutons, and remaining Parmesan cheese, then add the dressing and toss to coat. Serve.

Keeps for 1 day in the refrigerator.

ITALIAN BREAD SALAD

If you have leftover bread, or there is a sale on a good 100% whole grain loaf at the store, make this tasty salad. Toasted chunks of bread soak up the summery goodness of tomatoes, and fresh herbs pile on the flavor. If you already have a stash of croutons, just use four cups and skip making them again.

SERVES 8

4 cups cubed whole wheat bread (4 ounces)

2 tablespoons extra-virgin olive oil

2 garlic cloves, chopped

1 tablespoon fresh thyme leaves, chopped

½ teaspoon salt

½ teaspoon freshly ground black pepper

¼ cup shredded Parmesan cheese

2 cups grape tomatoes, halved

1 medium cucumber, peeled, seeded, and sliced

1 cup fresh parsley leaves, coarsely chopped

1 cup fresh basil leaves, coarsely chopped

DRESSING

1 garlic clove, pressed

3 tablespoons red wine vinegar

1 teaspoon granulated sugar

½ teaspoon salt

½ teaspoon freshly ground black pepper

¼ cup extra-virgin olive oil

Preheat the oven to 325°F.

Put the bread cubes in a large bowl. In a large sauté pan, heat the olive oil and sauté the garlic just until it sizzles, then add the thyme and stir briefly. Take off the heat and stir in the salt and the pepper. Pour the oil mixture over the bread cubes and toss to coat. Spread on a sheet pan and bake for 30 minutes. Stir, then sprinkle the Parmesan over the cubes and bake for 10 minutes more. Cool on a rack.

In a large bowl, combine the tomatoes, cucumber, parsley, and basil.

For the dressing, in a cup, whisk together the pressed garlic clove, vinegar, sugar, salt, pepper, and olive oil. Pour the dressing over the tomato mixture and toss to coat. Just before serving, toss with the bread cubes. The longer the salad stands, the softer the bread becomes. Best served the day it's made.

BUDDHA BOWLS FOR TWO

The "Buddha Bowl" is a lovely composition of grains, veggies, and healthy vegetarian foods, all placed on a big plate and drizzled with an Asian-inspired dressing. Keeping everything in separate piles allows you to enjoy many different tastes and textures, all while enjoying a complete meal.

SERVES 2

½ cup cooked red or black rice

4 handfuls baby kale mix or other salad greens, torn

2 pinches microgreens or pea sprouts

4 slices prebaked tofu, 1 cup cooked beans, or 1 scoop hummus

4 slices pickled beets, or ½ cup sauerkraut

½ medium avocado, sliced

2 large radishes or a small cucumber, slivered

1-inch piece fresh ginger, peeled and slivered

2 tablespoons pumpkin seeds or other seeds or nuts, toasted

DRESSING

2 tablespoons tahini

1 tablespoon soy sauce

2 tablespoons freshly squeezed lemon juice

1 tablespoon toasted sesame oil

2 tablespoons honey

1 teaspoon Sriracha sauce

If you are using leftover rice, warm it with a few drops of water in a small pan on the stove or in a bowl in the microwave.

Start building your bowls in two wide, shallow pasta-type bowls or on large dinner plates. Place the greens in the center and pile the microgreens on top. Around the greens, make piles of warm grain, tofu, beets, avocado, and radishes. Sprinkle slivered ginger on top of the greens and sprinkle pumpkin seeds on the piles of toppings.

For the dressing, in a cup, stir the tahini and soy sauce together with a fork until smooth, then stir in the lemon juice, sesame oil, honey, and Sriracha sauce to taste.

Drizzle the dressing over the bowls or serve it in a small dipping bowl to use as you eat.

MIXED RICE COBB _with_ AVOCADOS, BLUE CHEESE, AND CREAMY TOMATO DRESSING

If you want to make a salad appealing, make it as colorful and varied as this Cobb. It only takes a moment to compose it into a photo-ready spread, giving a hearty and healthy meal even more appeal.

SERVES 3 TO 4 AS A MAIN DISH, 4 TO 6 AS A SIDE DISH

½ cup brown rice blend, wheat berries, or other grain
   (or 1½ cups leftover cooked grain)

1 garlic clove, peeled

4 medium sun-dried tomatoes, rehydrated

1 tablespoon freshly squeezed lemon juice

¼ cup plain yogurt

1 tablespoon honey

¼ teaspoon salt

1 tablespoon extra-virgin olive oil

2 scallions, chopped (white and green parts)

1 heart of romaine lettuce, chopped

1 cup cherry tomatoes, sliced

1 large avocado, diced

2 ounces blue cheese, crumbled

1 large carrot, shredded

½ cup sunflower seeds, toasted

Cook your grain of choice, then let it cool in a medium bowl. In a food processor, mince the garlic and sun-dried tomatoes together. Add the lemon juice, yogurt, honey, salt, and olive oil and process until smooth, stopping to scrape down as necessary. Transfer the dressing to a cup (you should have about ¹/₂ cup).

   Add the scallions and half of the dressing to the bowl with the cooked grain and stir to mix.

   Spread the romaine on a large platter. Spoon the grain mixture over the lettuce to cover. Starting on one side of the platter, arrange rows of tomato, avocado, blue cheese, and carrot.

   Just before serving, drizzle the remaining dressing back and forth across the platter, sprinkle with the sunflower seeds, and place on the table. If desired, toss before serving, or allow diners to use tongs to serve themselves from the composed platter.

ROASTED CAULIFLOWER, CARROTS, AND PARMESAN CROUTONS OVER SPINACH

When it's cold outside, adding some cooked vegetables to salads just feels right. Roasting cauliflower and carrots gives them an appealing sweetness and concentrates their flavors to their essence. Crunchy croutons, tender spinach, and tangy dressing give this salad tons of texture and variety in every bite.

SERVES 4

2 cups Parmesan or plain croutons (page 70)

4 cups (12 ounces) large cauliflower florets

3 large carrots, cut into 1-inch chunks

4 garlic cloves, peeled

5 tablespoons extra-virgin olive oil, divided

1 ounce feta cheese (use a creamy-style feta, such as French sheep's milk feta)

2 tablespoons plain yogurt

½ teaspoon freshly ground black pepper

½ teaspoon salt

4 cups (4 ounces) fresh baby spinach

Prepare the croutons and reserve.

Preheat the oven to 400°F. In a large roasting pan, toss the cauliflower, carrots, and garlic cloves with 1 tablespoon of the olive oil. Cover the pan with a lid, a baking sheet, or aluminum foil and roast the vegetables for 20 minutes. Uncover the pan and roast for 10 minutes more to brown. Let cool. Pick out the garlic cloves for the dressing.

In a medium bowl, mash the feta with the roasted garlic. Stir in the yogurt, remaining olive oil, pepper, and salt. In a large bowl, combine the cauliflower mixture, croutons, spinach, and dressing and toss to coat well. Serve immediately.

SPINACH QUATTRO SALAD— FOUR SALADS ON ONE PLATE

People love options, don't they? If you are feeding a family of four, try this big platter topped with four takes on a grain salad. Give everyone a little of each and let them compare and contrast and pick their favorite. By the time the votes are in, the salad will be a happy memory, and everyone will be full of healthy whole grains and veggies.

SERVES 4

4 cups (4 ounces) fresh baby spinach leaves

3 cups cooked wheat berries or other grain
  (about 1 cup uncooked), divided

$\frac{1}{2}$ cup plain yogurt

$\frac{1}{2}$ teaspoon salt, divided

1 tablespoon honey

1 medium apple, chopped

$\frac{1}{4}$ cup crumbled blue cheese

2 tablespoons chopped fresh parsley

2 tablespoons extra-virgin olive oil

1 tablespoon Champagne vinegar

1 large tomato, cut into wedges

$\frac{1}{4}$ cup fresh basil leaves, julienned

$\frac{1}{2}$ cup corn kernels (thawed if frozen)

1 medium scallion, chopped (white and green parts)

Freshly ground black pepper

Distribute the spinach evenly among four medium-sized dinner plates. Put half of the grain in a medium bowl and stir in the yogurt and $\frac{1}{4}$ teaspoon of the salt. Transfer half of this mixture to another bowl and stir in the honey and apple; portion onto a quadrant of each plate. To the remaining grain-yogurt mixture, add the blue cheese and parsley, toss to combine, and portion onto another quadrant of each plate.

In a cup, whisk together the olive oil, vinegar, and remaining $\frac{1}{4}$ teaspoon salt. Combine the vinaigrette with the remaining cooked grain. Transfer half of this mixture to another bowl and mix in the tomato and basil; portion onto an empty quadrant of each plate. To the remaining grain-vinaigrette mixture, add the corn and scallion, toss to combine, and portion onto the remaining quadrant. Grind pepper over the salads and serve immediately.

WHEAT BERRY AND SHREDDED CABBAGE SALAD *WITH* BUTTERMILK DRESSING

Cabbage slaw seems to be relegated to summer picnics, but cabbage salads deserve a fresh take the rest of the year. This tangy, crunchy salad makes good use of that big head you picked up for soup, which is always a bargain and keeps for weeks in the crisper drawer. Just cook up some wheat berries and you have a salad that keeps for a few days, making this perfect for packing for lunch.

SERVES 4

1 cup spelt or wheat berries

4 cups water

1 garlic clove, pressed

1 large scallion, minced (white and green parts)

⅛ teaspoon cayenne pepper

1 teaspoon Dijon mustard

½ teaspoon salt

2 tablespoons mayonnaise

3 tablespoons plain Greek yogurt

¼ cup buttermilk

10 ounces green cabbage, slivered (4 cups)

1 large carrot, shredded

Boil the grain in the water, pasta-style, for 40 minutes to 1 hour. When the grain is tender to the bite, drain well and let cool.

In a medium cup, whisk together the garlic, scallion, cayenne, Dijon, salt, mayonnaise, yogurt, and buttermilk.

In a large bowl, combine the cooked grain, cabbage, and carrot. Pour the dressing over the grain mixture and toss to coat. Serve or store in an airtight container.

Keeps for 1 week in the refrigerator.

MIDDLE EASTERN FREEKEH SALAD
WITH SESAME-YOGURT DRESSING

Green wheat freekeh is the grain to watch, now that people have discovered its nutty, slightly toasted flavor. Because the wheat is harvested "green" and then roasted before hulling, chopping, and drying, freekeh has a deep flavor that you will love. Try it in this salad, with creamy yogurt dressing and little surprises like dates and olives in every bite.

SERVES 4 TO 6 (MAKES 6 CUPS)

1 cup freekeh, bulgur, or brown rice
1 cup fresh parsley leaves
½ cup fresh mint leaves
2 tablespoons honey
2 tablespoons tahini
½ cup plain Greek yogurt
2 tablespoons freshly squeezed lemon juice
2 tablespoons extra-virgin olive oil
1 teaspoon salt
1 medium cucumber, peeled, seeded, and chopped
½ cup pitted dates, sliced
½ cup Kalamata olives, sliced

Cook the grain according to the chart on page 20. Bring the required amount of water to a boil and add the grain. Return to a boil, cover tightly, then reduce the heat to the lowest setting. Cook, covered, for the suggested time. When all the water is absorbed, take the grain off the heat and let stand, covered, to steam for 5 minutes. Uncover and fluff to cool. Let cool completely. Can be made ahead and chilled.

Put the parsley and mint in the bowl of a food processor and mince, or mince the herbs by hand and place in a bowl. Add the honey, tahini, yogurt, lemon juice, olive oil, and salt and process or stir to mix.

Transfer the cooled grain to a large bowl and pour in the dressing, then add the cucumber, dates, and olives. Toss to mix, and serve.

Keeps for 3 days, tightly covered, in the refrigerator.

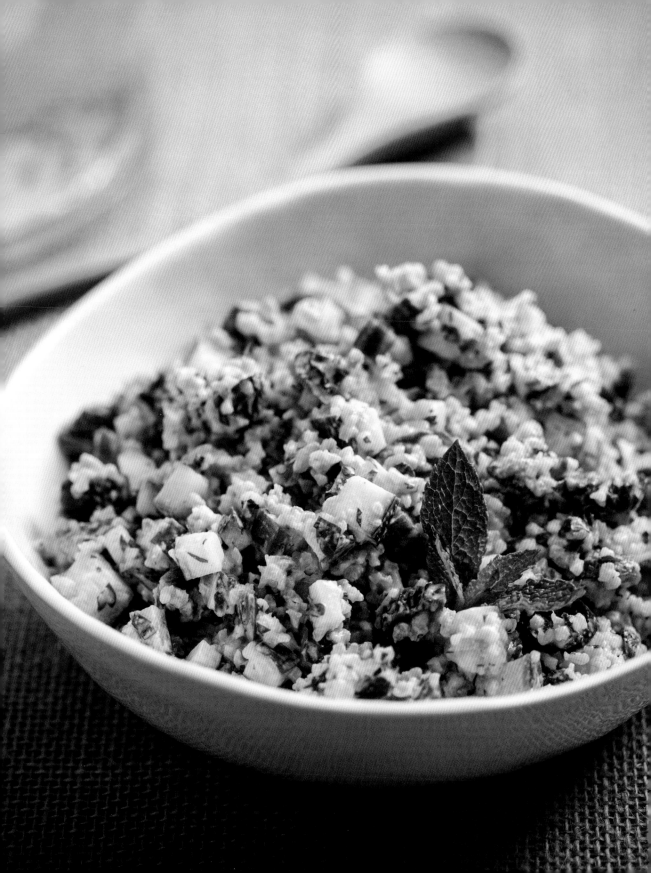

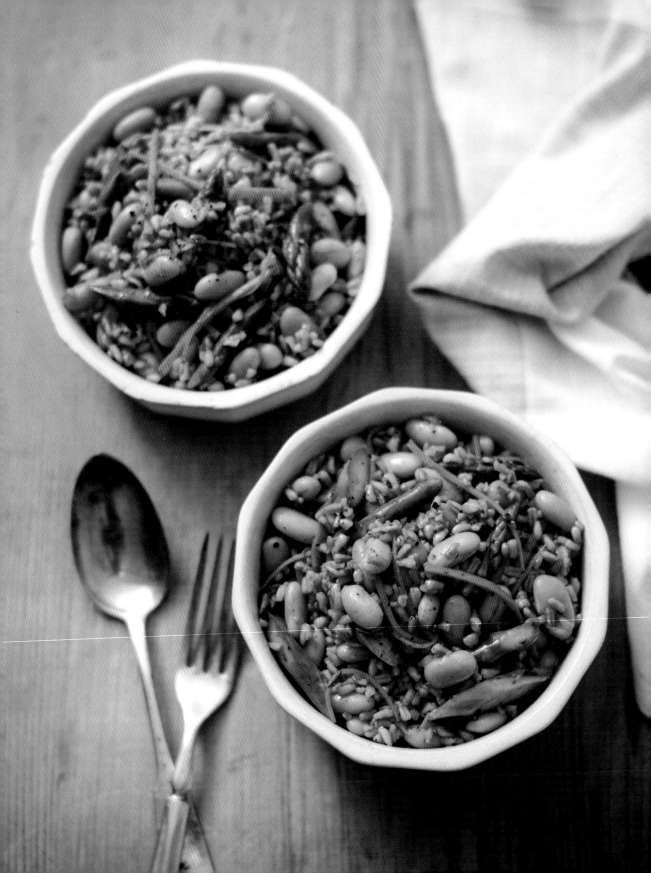

ITALIAN FARRO *and* WHITE BEAN SALAD WITH ASPARAGUS

Farro is old-school Italian and adds a crunchy contrast to the smooth and creamy white beans in this classic salad. This makes a scene-stealing side for simple roasted meats at dinner, or a wonderfully filling lunch all on its own. Feel free to substitute wheat berries, spelt, or even barley for the farro.

SERVES 4 TO 6 (MAKES 6 CUPS)

1 cup farro, spelt, or barley

4 cups water

½ bunch (8 ounces) asparagus, trimmed and cut into 2-inch pieces

1 small carrot, julienned

1½ cups cooked or canned cannellini beans, drained and rinsed

2 garlic cloves, crushed

2 tablespoons balsamic vinegar

1 tablespoon Dijon mustard

1 teaspoon fresh rosemary leaves, chopped

Pinch of sugar

½ teaspoon salt

¼ cup extra-virgin olive oil

In a 1-quart pot, boil the grain in the water, pasta-style, for about 40 minutes, depending on the grain (see the chart on page 20). When tender to the bite, drain and let cool.

Set up a steamer and steam the asparagus and carrot for 1 minute; they should still be crisp. Drain and pat dry on a kitchen towel.

In a large bowl, combine the cooked grain, asparagus and carrot, and beans. In a cup, whisk together the garlic, vinegar, mustard, rosemary, sugar, and salt. Whisk in the olive oil and pour over the grain mixture. Toss to coat and serve at room temperature.

Keeps for 4 days, tightly covered, in the refrigerator.

SUSHI BROCCOLI *AND* BROWN RICE SALAD

Sushi is no longer exotic, now that we have embraced vinegary rice and spicy wasabi and absorbed it into our national palate. Here, a salad with all the flavors you love in sushi can answer that craving with very little effort. You can make a heartier meal of it by roasting some tofu, fish, or chicken with teriyaki sauce to place on top.

SERVES 6 TO 8 (MAKES ABOUT 8 CUPS)

1 cup short-grain brown, black, or red rice

2 cups water

3 tablespoons rice vinegar

2 tablespoons granulated sugar

1 tablespoon canola oil

½ teaspoon salt

3 cups large broccoli florets (from 1 stalk)

5-inch piece (10 ounces) daikon, peeled and julienned

¼ cup pickled ginger, chopped

1 avocado

3 medium scallions, sliced on a diagonal (white and green parts)

Nori seaweed, slivered with kitchen scissors

In a 1-quart pot, bring the rice and water to a boil. Cover tightly and reduce the heat to low. Cook for 35 to 40 minutes, or until all the water is absorbed. Take the pan off the heat and let stand, covered, for at least 5 minutes before scraping the rice into a large bowl.

While the rice is still warm, stir together the vinegar, sugar, canola oil, and salt in a cup and pour over the rice. Gently fold in the dressing to coat the grains without breaking them.

Prepare the broccoli, if desired (you can steam the broccoli for a minute, just until crisp-tender), or leave it raw. Add the broccoli, daikon, and ginger to the rice and toss to mix. Just before serving, cut the avocado in half and remove the pit, then slice the avocado while still in the shell and scoop out the slices with a spoon. Top the salad with avocado, scallions, and nori and serve immediately.

To serve later, wait to slice and add the avocado, scallions, and nori until just before serving. The untopped salad keeps for 4 days, tightly covered, in the refrigerator.

SOBA OR WHOLE WHEAT SPAGHETTI WITH SESAME DRESSING AND SUGAR SNAP PEAS

There is something perfect and fascinating about the combination of flavors in a good sesame noodle. Roasted, rich sesame paste, combined with salty, fermented soy sauce and tart vinegar creates a dressing that you will want to slather on everything. Simple buckwheat or whole wheat noodles and crunchy sugar snap peas carry it well.

SERVES 6 (MAKES ABOUT 7 CUPS)

¼ cup tahini

1 garlic clove, minced or crushed

1 tablespoon chopped fresh ginger

2 tablespoons soy sauce

2 tablespoons brewed tea or water

1 tablespoon rice vinegar

1 tablespoon honey

7 ounces sugar snap peas, trimmed

1 large carrot, julienned

8 ounces 100% buckwheat soba noodles or whole wheat fettuccine

2 large scallions, slivered (white and green parts)

1 small cucumber, peeled, seeded, and sliced

Sriracha sauce, for serving

Put on a large pot of well-salted water to boil for the pasta. In a cup, stir together the tahini, garlic, ginger, soy sauce, and tea. When smooth, stir in the rice vinegar and honey. Reserve.

Put the trimmed snap peas and julienned carrot in the colander that you will drain the pasta in.

Cook the pasta according to package directions, about 9 minutes to al dente. Drain, pouring the boiling water and pasta over the veggies in the colander. Shake to drain thoroughly. Place the pasta, snap peas, and carrot in a large bowl, drizzle with the tahini mixture, and toss. Top with the scallions and cucumber at serving, or mix them in and refrigerate for later. Pass Sriracha sauce for diners to add to taste, or drizzle decoratively over the noodles on a platter.

Keeps for 4 days, tightly covered, in the refrigerator.

LIME QUINOA SALAD
WITH AVOCADO AND MANGO

Quinoa is excellent in chilled salads, with its delicate texture that stays tender even when cold. Bright orange mango and creamy green avocado chunks make this simple salad pop—both on the plate and in your mouth!

SERVES 4 (MAKES 4½ CUPS)

1½ cups water

1 cup quinoa

¼ cup freshly squeezed lime juice

1 teaspoon freshly grated lime zest

½ teaspoon salt

¼ cup canola oil

½ cup fresh cilantro leaves, coarsely chopped

1 medium red jalapeño pepper, seeded and chopped

1 large carrot, shredded

1 large mango, peeled and chopped

1 large avocado, cubed

2 medium scallions, chopped (white and green parts)

In a 1-quart pot, bring the water to a boil and add the quinoa. Return to a boil, reduce the heat to low, and cover tightly. Cook for about 14 minutes, or until all the water is absorbed. Take off the heat and let cool.

In a cup, whisk together the lime juice, zest, salt, and canola oil. Pour over the cooled quinoa.

Transfer the quinoa to a large bowl and add the cilantro, jalapeño, carrot, mango, avocado, and scallions. Toss to mix and serve.

Keeps for 1 day, tightly covered, in the refrigerator. To make a few days ahead, wait to add the avocado and mango until just before serving.

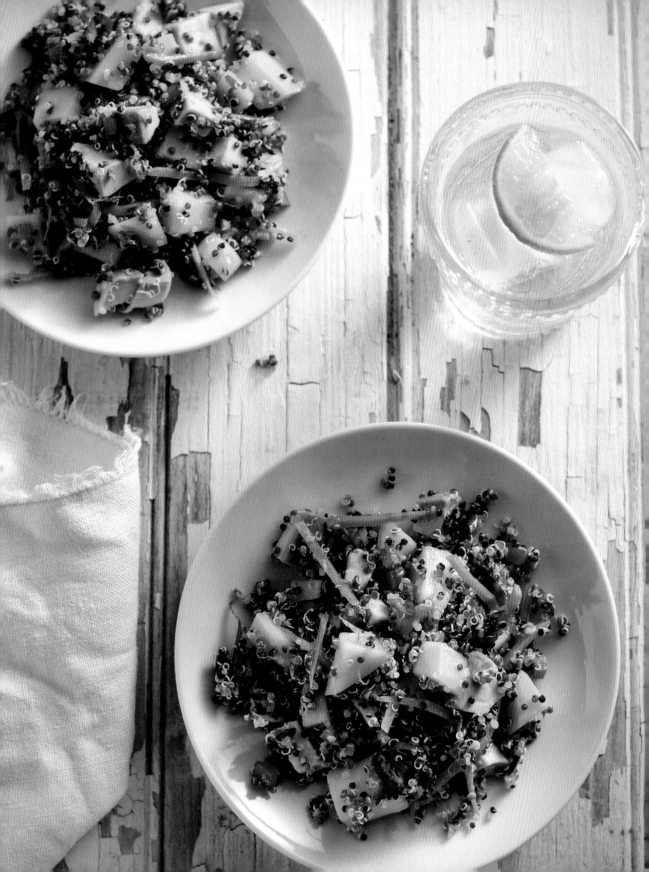

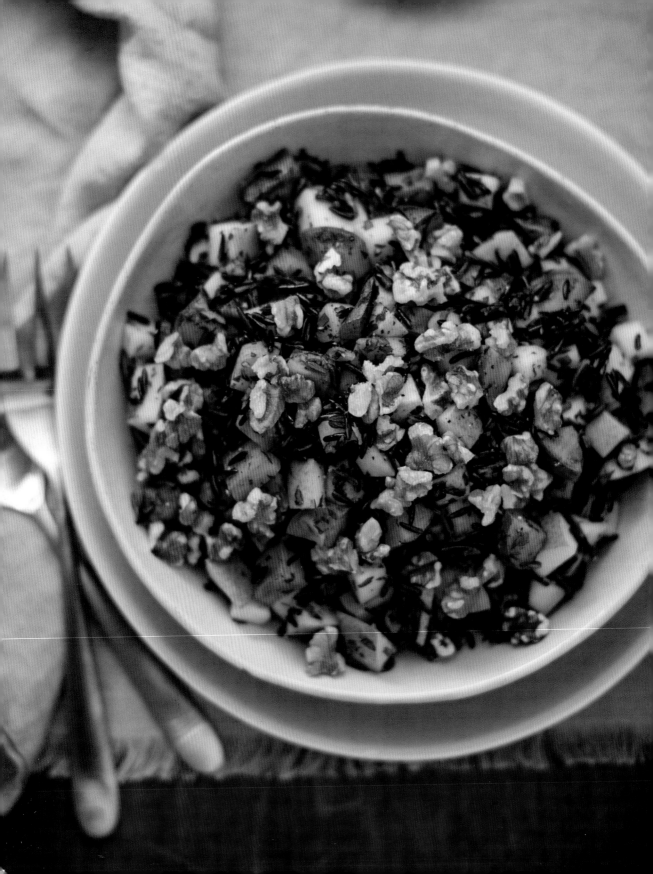

WILD RICE, PEAR, *and* ROASTED SWEET POTATO SALAD WITH WALNUTS

In the colder months, take a break from your usual mashed potatoes or yams and try this sweet and savory treat. Wild rice has a deep flavor that has given it a gourmet reputation, in spite of the healthfulness of the grain. If you can find true hand-harvested wild rice from the Great Lakes region, you absolutely must splurge and show off your acquisition in this delicious salad.

SERVES 6 (MAKES ABOUT 7 CUPS)

3 cups water
1 cup wild rice or a rice blend
1 pound sweet potato, cubed (4 cups)
4 tablespoons extra-virgin olive oil, divided
½ cup fresh parsley leaves, chopped
2 large scallions, chopped (white and green parts)
2 medium ripe pears, cored and chopped
¼ cup freshly squeezed lemon juice
2 tablespoons Grade B maple syrup
½ teaspoon salt
½ teaspoon freshly ground black pepper
½ cup walnut pieces, coarsely chopped

First, cook the wild rice. Truly wild rice and cultivated wild rice have very different cooking times. Add the water to a 2-quart pot and bring to a boil. Add the rice and return to a boil, then reduce the heat to a simmer and cover the pot. For hand-harvested wild rice, start checking in 20 minutes. Cultivated rice may take 45 minutes to 1 hour. When the rice is tender and just starting to split apart at the ends, drain well. Let cool.

Preheat the oven to 400°F. On a large sheet pan, toss the sweet potatoes with 1 tablespoon of the olive oil. Roast for 20 minutes, stir, and then roast for 10 minutes more, depending on the size of your cubes. When the cubes are easily pierced with a paring knife, they are done. Let cool to room temperature.

In a large bowl, combine the wild rice, sweet potatoes, parsley, scallions, and pears. In a small bowl, whisk together the remaining olive oil, lemon juice, maple syrup, salt, and pepper. Pour the dressing over the wild rice mixture and toss to coat.

Serve topped with walnuts.

Keeps for 2 to 3 days, tightly covered, in the refrigerator. If you want to store it longer, wait to chop the pears until just before serving.

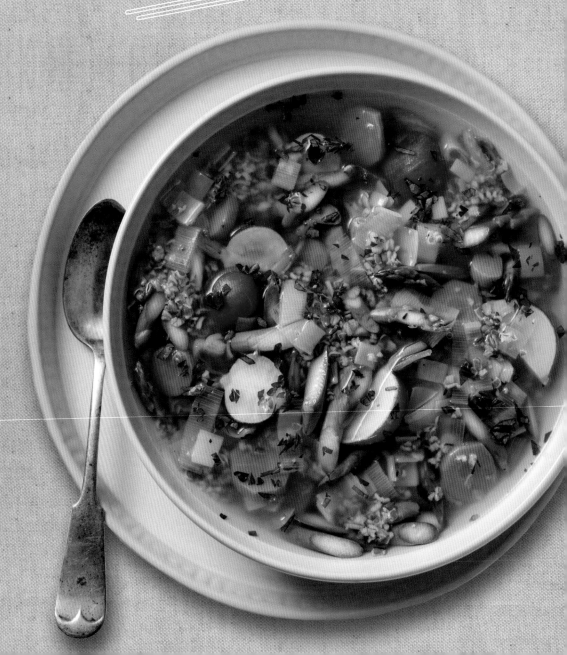

SOUPS

QUICK VEGGIE CHILI
WITH MUSHROOMS AND BULGUR

Why bother with ground beef, when you can get a deep, meaty flavor from minced mushrooms and bulgur, with no cholesterol or saturated fat? Bulgur has been the go-to grain for veggie chili for years, since the chewy bits are about the same size as bits of ground beef, and the thirsty grain drinks up the flavorful liquids of the chili, making it thick and hearty. Use a beer that is pale or amber—not too hoppy. You can drink one with the chili, too.

SERVES 6 (MAKES ABOUT 6 CUPS)

2 teaspoons extra-virgin olive oil

1 medium onion, chopped

1 large carrot, chopped

8 ounces button mushrooms, washed and dried

4 teaspoons chili powder

½ teaspoon chipotle powder

1 cup vegetable stock

¾ cup beer, divided

1 teaspoon Worcestershire sauce (regular or vegan)

½ cup bulgur

1 (14½-ounce) can fire-roasted tomato purée

1 medium red bell pepper, chopped

1 medium green bell pepper, chopped

1 (15-ounce) can black beans, with juice (or 1½ cups cooked black beans)

1 teaspoon dried oregano

½ teaspoon salt

¼ cup tomato paste

In a large pot, heat the olive oil over medium heat and sauté the onion and carrot for 5 minutes, or until soft. In a food processor, pulse the mushrooms to mince, not purée, then scrape into the pot. Raise the heat to medium high to sear and soften the mushrooms; cook for about 5 minutes.

Add the chili powder and chipotle powder and stir until fragrant, then add the vegetable stock, ½ cup of the beer, Worcestershire, bulgur, and tomato purée and stir. Raise the heat to high and bring to a boil, then cover and reduce to medium-low. Simmer for 20 minutes. Uncover and add the red and green peppers, black beans, oregano, and salt, stirring to combine. In a cup, stir the remaining beer with the tomato paste and then stir that into the pot. Simmer for another 5 to 10 minutes to combine the flavors and thicken the chili. Serve.

Keeps for 1 week, tightly covered, in the refrigerator.

CREAMY CURRIED CARROT-MILLET SOUP *with* MINT

If creamy soups intimidate you, try this easy purée. Sunny yellow millet cooks to melting softness, then gets puréed with the carrots, creating a thick, creamy soup with no flour and no cream necessary. You can make it as thick or as thin as you like by adding more or less milk.

SERVES 4

1 tablespoon canola oil
1 medium onion, chopped
2 teaspoons curry powder
Pinch of cayenne pepper
4 large carrots, chopped (15 ounces/2½ cups)
½ cup millet
3 cups chicken or vegetable stock, plus water as needed
1 cup whole milk
½ teaspoon salt
1 cup plain yogurt, for garnish
½ cup fresh mint leaves, sliced

Place a 2-quart saucepan over medium heat, and when hot, add the oil. Add the onion and sauté until softened, then lower the heat and cook slowly until golden, about 10 minutes. Add the curry powder, cayenne, carrots, and millet and stir until fragrant. Add the stock, bring to a boil, and reduce the heat to the lowest setting. Cover and cook for 40 minutes. (Check at 30 minutes and add water, if necessary, to keep the millet from sticking to the pot.)

Uncover the pot; the millet should be completely broken apart and porridge-like. Transfer the contents of the pot to a food processor or blender. Use a folded kitchen towel to cover the top and hold the lid, then purée the mixture thoroughly, taking care not to burn yourself. Gradually add the milk with the machine running. Add the salt and pulse to mix.

Scrape the soup back into the pot to reheat or hold until serving time.

Serve each bowl garnished with ¼ cup yogurt and some fresh mint.

Keeps for 1 week, tightly covered, in the refrigerator.

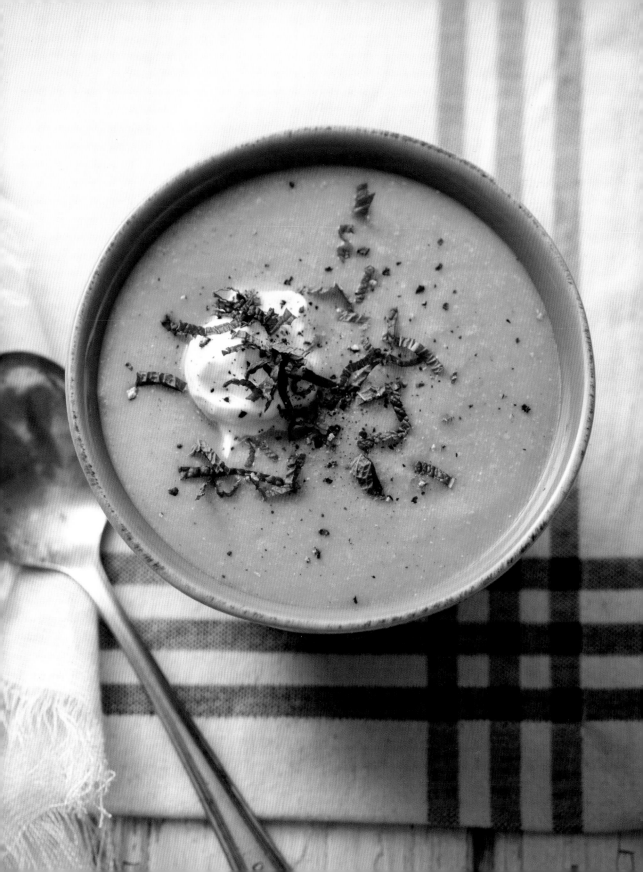

CREAMY SPINACH SOUP

Prewashed, bagged spinach has made healthy cooking so much easier. Just a quick rinse and you have a leafy green that cooks in a snap. In this deep-green soup, spinach goes for a spin with whole grains for a tasty and comforting soup. For a beautiful meal, serve a cup of the green soup nestled alongside vibrant red Whole Wheat Penne in Roasted-Pepper Romesco Sauce (page 116).

SERVES 4 (MAKES ABOUT 4 CUPS)

1 tablespoon unsalted butter
1 large onion, chopped
½ cup short-grain brown rice, millet, or amaranth
1½ cups water
1 bay leaf
½ teaspoon salt
2 (5-ounce) bags fresh spinach, or 10 ounces
   bulk fresh spinach leaves, divided
1 cup milk, plus more as needed

In a large pot, melt the butter and sauté the onion over medium heat. Cook, stirring often, for about 10 minutes. When soft and golden, add the grain, water, and bay leaf and raise the heat to bring to a boil. Cover and cook for the recommended time for that grain (see the chart on page 20), plus about 5 minutes. You want the grain very soft. Remove the bay leaf.

When the grain is cooked, add the salt and two thirds of the spinach. Cover and let the heat wilt the leaves, about 5 minutes over low. Transfer the contents of the pot to a blender or food processor, being careful not to burn yourself.

Purée the soup until creamy, adding milk as you go. Chop the remaining spinach. Scrape the soup back into the pot and heat. Stir in the chopped spinach and cook just until softened. Add more milk, if desired.

Serve warm or let cool and store.

Keeps for 4 days, tightly covered, in the refrigerator.

FAST CHICKEN SOUP _with_ QUINOA

With boxed stock and some boneless, skinless chicken, you can have chicken soup on the table in minutes, not hours. Quinoa is a perfect grain for soup, cooking quickly and adding both flavor and a protein boost, but you can always try this method with other grains, too.

SERVES 4 (MAKES ABOUT 5 CUPS)

1 tablespoon extra-virgin olive oil

1 large onion, chopped

1 large carrot, chopped

4 cups chicken stock

1 cup water

½ cup millet, quinoa, freekeh, or brown rice

½ teaspoon salt

½ teaspoon freshly ground black pepper

1 large (8-ounce) chicken breast, chopped into bite-sized pieces

1 teaspoon dried thyme

2 cups greens, such as spinach, chard, or kale, stemmed and coarsely chopped

In a 4-quart pot, heat the olive oil over medium-high heat. Add the onion and carrot and sauté for 5 minutes, or until the onion is soft and golden. Pour in the stock, water, and grain, stir in the salt and pepper, and bring to a boil. Cover, turn the heat to low, and cook for the amount of time recommended for your chosen grain (see the chart on page 20; 15 minutes for quinoa, 25 for millet, etc.).

When the grain is tender, uncover and raise the heat to medium, then add the chicken and thyme and simmer until the chicken is cooked through, about 5 minutes. Stir in the greens and cook until wilted. Take off the heat and serve hot, or cool completely and store.

Keeps for 4 days, tightly covered, in the refrigerator.

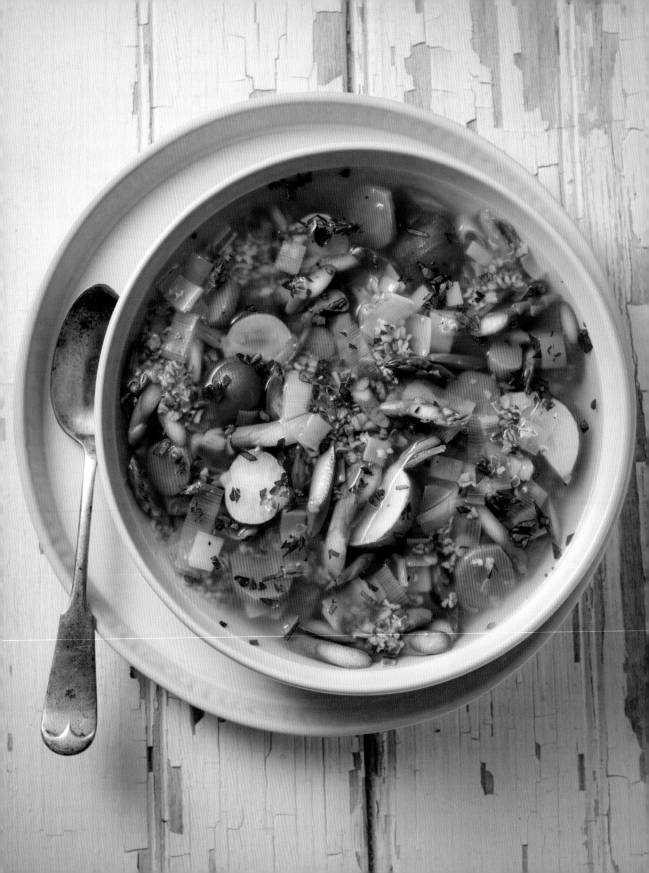

SPRING VEGGIE STEW ᴡ͟ɪᴛ͟ʜ BULGUR

Celebrate spring by making this delicious soup, full of the freshest veggies and chewy bulgur. Veggie and grain soups are a great way to fill up and stay satisfied, with a minimum of calories and lots of plant-based nutrition. Serve a bowl to start the meal and you're likely to eat less of everything else.

SERVES 6 (MAKES ABOUT 8 CUPS)

1 tablespoon extra-virgin olive oil

2 large leeks, sliced and washed

4 large red radishes, quartered

1 medium carrot, chopped

1 tablespoon fresh thyme

1 large bay leaf

4 cups vegetable stock

2 cups water

½ cup bulgur

½ teaspoon salt

1 bunch (1 pound) asparagus, cut into 1-inch pieces

½ cup fresh parsley leaves, chopped

Heat a large pot over medium-high heat and add the olive oil. Add the leeks, radishes, carrot, and thyme. Lower the heat and sauté until the leeks are softened, stirring often. Add the bay leaf, stock, water, bulgur, and salt and bring to a simmer. Turn off the heat and let stand for 15 minutes. Remove the bay leaf. Add the asparagus and parsley and cook for 2 minutes to soften. Serve hot, or store. Keeps for 1 week, tightly covered, in the refrigerator.

BEET AND BUCKWHEAT BORSCHT
⟨WITH⟩ PARSLEY-YOGURT GARNISH

For the beet lover in you! Beets and buckwheat were made for each other, with earthy, undeniable flavors and textures that are complementary and so northern European. In this gorgeous presentation, the ruby red soup gets a floating mound of savory buckwheat and a green and white dollop of yogurt to really paint a delectable picture.

SERVES 6 TO 8

(MAKES ABOUT 8 CUPS)

½ cup buckwheat groats

¾ cup water

1 tablespoon extra-virgin olive oil

1 cup chopped onion

1 pound red beets, peeled and chopped (3 cups)

2 medium carrots, chopped

2 stalks celery, chopped

1 teaspoon caraway seeds

1 cup apple juice

3 cups water or stock

2 cups beet greens (or other leafy greens), washed and chopped

1 teaspoon salt

1 teaspoon dried dill

1 tablespoon red wine vinegar

GARNISH

¾ cup plain yogurt

½ cup fresh parsley leaves, chopped

¼ teaspoon salt

In a 1-quart pot with a tight-fitting lid, dry-toast the buckwheat over medium-high heat until fragrant. Carefully pour in the water, then bring to a boil. Cover tightly and turn the heat to low. Cook for 15 to 20 minutes, or until all the water is absorbed. Take the pan off the heat and keep warm until the soup is finished.

Put a large pot over high heat, and when hot, add the oil. Add the onion and sauté, lowering the heat when the onion starts to brown. Cook for an hour if you can; longer cooking will bring out the onion's sugars. Add the beets, carrots, and celery and keep stirring for about 5 minutes. Add the caraway, apple juice, water or stock, and beet greens and bring to a boil. Once boiling, lower to a simmer and cook until the beets are very tender, about 10 minutes. Add the salt, dill, and vinegar and simmer for another 5 minutes.

For the garnish, stir the yogurt with the parsley and salt.

To serve, ladle a cup of the soup in a wide soup bowl, then put a ¼-cup portion of buckwheat in the center and a tablespoon of the yogurt mixture on top. Serve immediately.

The three components keep for 1 week, tightly covered, in the refrigerator.

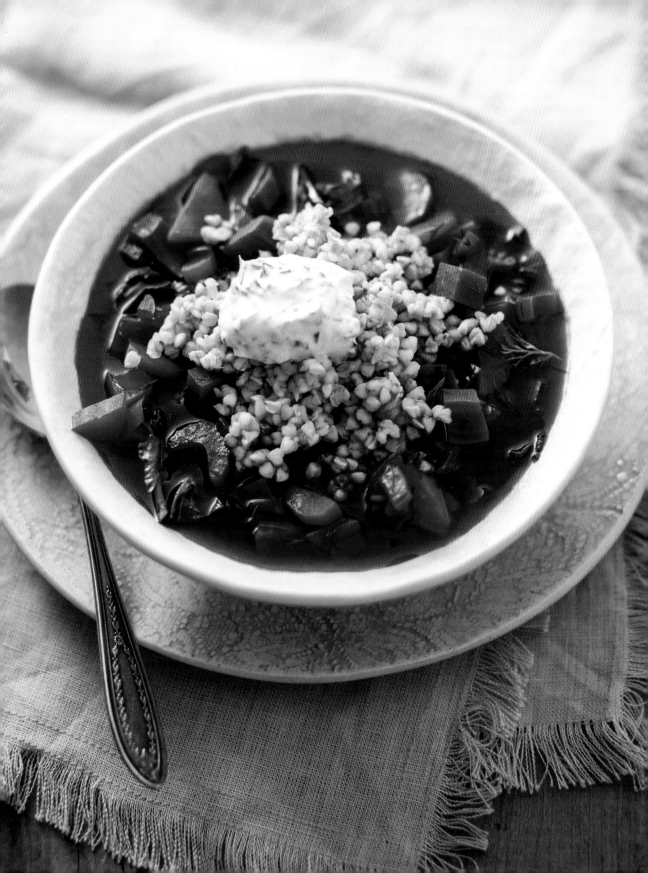

SUMMER TOMATO-ZUCCHINI SOUP
ᵂᴵᵀᴴ WHEAT BERRIES

When vine-ripened tomatoes are at their peak, and your neighbor with a garden can't use up all her crisp, sun-soaked zucchini, make this soup. Wheat berries make a delightful, slightly crunchy counterpoint to the tender veggies, or you can use a grain that will melt into the soup, like brown rice or barley. To make this even faster, use 1½ cups of leftover cooked barley, wild rice, or other favorite grain in place of the wheat berries.

SERVES 6 (MAKES ABOUT 8 CUPS)

3 cups water
½ cup wheat berries
1 tablespoon extra-virgin olive oil
1 large onion, chopped
2 garlic cloves, chopped
2 tablespoons fresh rosemary leaves, chopped
2 medium zucchini, quartered and sliced (3 cups)
4 medium tomatoes, chopped (3 cups)
½ cup white wine
2 cups chicken or vegetable stock
½ teaspoon salt
½ teaspoon freshly ground black pepper
1 cup fresh basil leaves, chopped

In a pot, bring the water and wheat berries to a boil, then reduce to a simmer and cook for 1 hour. Test for tenderness, drain when ready, and reserve.

Heat the olive oil in a 4-quart pot over medium-high heat. Add the onion and sauté, stirring, for about 5 minutes. Reduce the heat and add the garlic and rosemary, stirring for 1 to 2 minutes, or until fragrant. Add the zucchini and tomatoes and turn the heat up to high, stirring until the tomatoes are juicy and the zucchini starts to brown a little. Add the wine, stock, salt, and pepper and bring to a boil, then reduce the heat to simmer gently. Add the cooked grain and simmer to heat through.

Stir in the basil just before serving. Keeps for 1 week, tightly covered, in the refrigerator.

MILLET-CORN CHOWDER WITH CHIPOTLE

Sweet and summery corn and soft yellow millet make a sunny chowder, and, spiked with bright red peppers, this colorful soup will please your eye as much as your palate. A smoky, spicy hit of chipotle takes it to another level of deliciousness.

SERVES 4 (MAKES ABOUT 4 CUPS)

2 teaspoons olive oil

1 large onion, chopped

½ cup millet

2 cups water

1 (10-ounce) package frozen corn, or 2 ears
   fresh corn (kernels cut off the cob), divided

2 cups milk

1 teaspoon salt

½ teaspoon freshly ground black pepper

½ teaspoon ground chipotle pepper

½ cup fresh parsley leaves, chopped

½ cup chopped red bell pepper

In a large pot, heat the oil over medium heat. Add the onion and sauté for at least 5 minutes, or until golden. Add the millet and water and bring to a boil. Cover, reduce the heat to low, and cook for 25 minutes, or until the millet is very soft. Transfer the mixture to a food processor or blender and add half of the corn. Carefully purée, stopping to scrape down as necessary, and adding milk as you go to make a smooth mixture.

Transfer the corn purée back into the soup pot. Stir in the remaining corn and the salt, pepper, chipotle, parsley, and red bell pepper. Over medium heat, bring to a simmer, but don't boil too vigorously. Cook until the pepper is softened, then serve warm.

Keeps for 1 week, tightly covered, in the refrigerator.

MEXICAN TORTILLA SOUP *with* SHRIMP

Whole grain tortillas, sliced and baked to make crispy strips, are the Mexican version of saltines in a savory soup like this one. Wait to float the strips in the soup until just before serving so that they will stay crunchy as you enjoy the soup.

SERVES 6 TO 8 (MAKES 8 CUPS)

1 tablespoon extra-virgin olive oil

1 large onion, chopped

2 garlic cloves, chopped

Pinch of ground cloves

1 teaspoon ground cumin

½ teaspoon ground chipotle pepper

1 teaspoon dried oregano

1 medium zucchini, diced

1 small red bell pepper, chopped

4 cups vegetable or chicken stock

¾ teaspoon salt, divided

8 ounces peeled and deveined shrimp, chopped

5 (7-inch) corn tortillas (preferably the stone-ground, very yellow ones)

1 tablespoon canola oil

½ teaspoon chili powder

½ cup fresh cilantro leaves, for garnish

1 large lime, cut into wedges, for serving

In a large pot, heat the olive oil over high heat and add the onion. Lower the heat to medium and stir for 5 minutes or so, or until the onion softens, then add the garlic, ground cloves, cumin, chipotle, and oregano. Stir for a few seconds. Add the zucchini and red bell pepper and stir for a few minutes, then pour in the stock and bring to a boil. Add ½ teaspoon of the salt. Reduce the heat to a simmer and cook for about 10 minutes. Stir in the shrimp and cook just until pink, then take the pot off the heat and keep warm.

Preheat the oven to 375°F. Stack the tortillas and slice into ¼-inch strips. Place them on a baking sheet and drizzle with the canola oil, chili powder, and remaining ¼ teaspoon salt. Bake for 20 to 25 minutes, stirring every 5 minutes, or until the strips are crisp.

Garnish the soup with the cilantro and tortilla strips and serve with lime wedges for squeezing over the soup.

The soup keeps for 3 days, tightly covered, in the refrigerator. The tortilla strips keep for 1 week in an airtight container at room temperature.

SPICY CABBAGE SOUP
WITH LEFTOVER-GRAIN DUMPLINGS

A steaming bowl of soup that is topped with tender, spoonable dumplings is the essence of comfort in a bowl. Cabbage is an inexpensive and incredibly healthy vegetable—the perfect backdrop for a filling and satisfying soup. Vegetarians can use a meatless sausage, if desired.

SERVES 6

1 tablespoon extra-virgin olive oil

4 ounces Italian sausage, crumbled

1 medium onion, chopped

12 ounces green cabbage, chopped (3 cups)

2 medium carrots, chopped

2 garlic cloves, chopped

2 cups chicken stock

1 (14½-ounce) can diced tomatoes, with juice

½ cup white wine

DUMPLINGS

½ cup white whole wheat flour

½ teaspoon baking soda

½ teaspoon salt

1 large egg

2 tablespoons buttermilk

½ cup cooked millet or other grain

Grated Parmesan cheese, for serving

In a large pot, heat the olive oil over medium-high heat and brown the sausage. Add the onion and cook until softened. Add the cabbage and carrot and stir until the cabbage is a little bit browned, about 5 minutes. Add the garlic and stir for a minute, then add the stock, tomatoes and their juice, and wine. Bring to a boil, then reduce the heat to simmer.

For the dumplings, while the stew simmers, in a large bowl, combine the flour, baking soda, and salt. In a cup, whisk together the egg and buttermilk, then stir into the flour mixture. When the flour is incorporated, stir in the cooked grain.

Drop tablespoon-sized portions of the dumpling dough onto the surface of the simmering stew, leaving a little space between them. Cover the pot and cook for 5 minutes. The dumplings should be puffed and solid to the touch.

Serve the stew with dumplings on top. Pass Parmesan on the side.

Keeps for 4 days, tightly covered, in the refrigerator.

SIDES

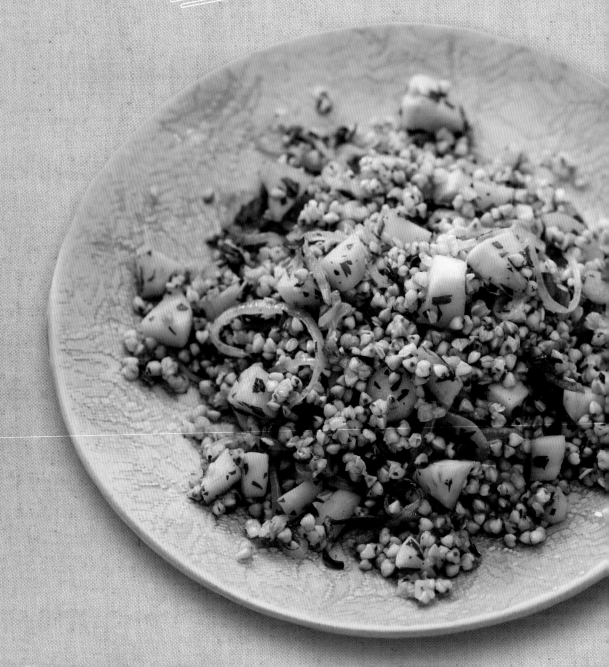

EASY BULGUR HERB PILAF

Pilafs are too often just oily, white-rice-based sides—bland and boring. This bulgur pilaf is bursting with nutty flavor and texture, and it cooks just as quickly as white rice. It's a perfect complement to meat, fish, or an herby bean dish.

SERVES 4 (MAKES ABOUT 4 CUPS)

1 teaspoon extra-virgin olive oil
1 small onion, chopped
1 large carrot, chopped
2 cups chicken or vegetable stock
1 teaspoon dried thyme
½ teaspoon salt
1¼ cups bulgur
½ cup fresh parsley leaves, chopped

In a 2-quart pot with a tight-fitting lid, heat the olive oil briefly over medium heat, then add the onion and carrot. Sauté until the onion is soft and translucent, about 5 minutes. Add the stock, thyme, and salt and bring to a boil. Add the bulgur and return to a boil, then reduce the heat to low. Cover and set a timer for 15 minutes.

Let stand, covered, for 5 more minutes to steam. Stir in the parsley and serve warm.

Keeps for 1 week, tightly covered, in the refrigerator.

QUICK LEMONY COUSCOUS WITH SPINACH

Whole wheat couscous is the all-time fast-grain champ, and most people will not even notice that your couscous is whole grain instead of white. In this quick side, vibrant lemon and tender spinach cook along with the tiny couscous grains, adding flavor and veggie goodness. Pair this with a Mediterranean-flavored main or a tub of hummus and veggie dippers.

SERVES 4 (MAKES ABOUT 4 CUPS)

2 teaspoons extra-virgin olive oil

2 garlic cloves, chopped

2 medium scallions, chopped (white and green parts)

1 lemon wedge (¼ of a large lemon)

1 teaspoon dried thyme

¼ teaspoon salt

1¼ cups vegetable stock

1 cup whole wheat couscous

4 cups (4 ounces) fresh spinach, chopped

In a 4-quart pot with a tight-fitting lid, heat the olive oil briefly over medium heat. Add the garlic and scallions and stir for 1 minute. Add the lemon wedge, thyme, and salt and stir for 1 minute. Pour in the stock, raise the heat to high, and bring to a boil. Once boiling, turn off the heat. Immediately dump in the couscous, give it a quick stir, and cover.

Let stand for 5 minutes. Quickly stir in the spinach and cover again for 5 minutes. Remove the lemon wedge. Serve hot.

Keeps for 1 week, tightly covered, in the refrigerator.

HERBED BREAD STUFFING

You don't have to wait for the holidays to enjoy the comforting sensation of warm, familiar stuffing. I've been known to freeze the odds and ends left over from loaves of bread, and when I have enough, bring them out for a batch of stuffing.

SERVES 6

1 tablespoon olive oil, plus more for the pan

1 medium onion, chopped

4 stalks celery, chopped

1 medium carrot, chopped

½ cup bulgur

2½ cups vegetable or chicken stock

½ teaspoon freshly ground black pepper

½ teaspoon dried thyme

2 teaspoons dried sage

1 teaspoon salt

4 cups cubed whole wheat bread

½ cup hazelnuts, toasted, skins rubbed off

Preheat the oven to 400°F and lightly oil a 2-quart baking pan. In a 4-quart pot, heat the olive oil and add the onion, celery, and carrot. Sauté for about 5 minutes to soften. Add the bulgur and stock and raise the heat to bring to a boil. Cover, lower the heat, and simmer for about 15 minutes.

Uncover and stir. Test the bulgur; it should be tender. Add the pepper, thyme, sage, and salt and stir, then fold in the bread cubes. Transfer the mixture to the prepared pan. Press into the pan and top with the hazelnuts, gently pressing the nuts into the surface of the stuffing.

Bake for about 20 minutes, or until crusty on top. Serve hot.

Once cooled, keeps for 1 week, tightly covered, in the refrigerator.

EASY BASIL BAKED POLENTA ROUNDS

Whole grain coarse-grind polenta is a great whole grain food, and it's a gorgeous yellow color to boot! Bake up these pretty biscuit-sized rounds of basil- and Parmesan-laced polenta and serve them as the pasta course or for a light lunch with a salad. For a grainy variation, try substituting half amaranth or millet for the polenta.

SERVES 9

2½ cups water

1 teaspoon salt

1 tablespoon unsalted butter, plus more for the pan

1 cup polenta or coarse cornmeal (substitute ½ cup with amaranth or millet, if desired)

½ cup fresh basil leaves, chopped

½ cup shredded Parmesan cheese

½ teaspoon freshly ground black pepper

Olive oil, for frying (optional)

Grease a 9-inch square baking pan and reserve. Bring the water, salt, and butter to a boil. Whisk in the polenta gradually. Reduce the heat and simmer for 30 to 40 minutes, stirring every 5 minutes.

When the polenta is tender and thick, stir in the basil, Parmesan, and pepper. Pour into the prepared pan, then smooth with a spatula. Chill, covered, until cold.

Use a 3-inch biscuit cutter to cut out rounds or simply cut 3 x 3 to make squares. Bake on an oiled baking sheet at 375°F for about 15 minutes or fry in olive oil over medium-high heat. Serve hot.

Keeps for 1 week, tightly covered, in the refrigerator.

WHOLE WHEAT ANGEL HAIR
WITH ARUGULA-RICOTTA PESTO

Whole wheat angel hair cooks in four minutes, and the thin noodles are almost indistinguishable from white pasta once you sauce them up and take a bite. In this quick and easy dish, ricotta adds some protein and subtle sweetness to the pesto. Arugula is easy to get year-round, and it makes a great pesto when basil is scarce and expensive.

SERVES 4 (MAKES 6 CUPS)

2 cups (6 ounces) broccoli or cauliflower florets
1 medium carrot, julienned
2 cups (2½ ounces) arugula leaves
1 garlic clove, peeled
½ teaspoon salt
2 tablespoons extra-virgin olive oil
½ cup part-skim ricotta cheese
¼ cup shredded Parmesan cheese
8 ounces whole wheat angel hair or spaghetti
1 cup chopped fresh tomatoes

Bring a big pot of salted water to a boil for the pasta. While it is heating, prepare the broccoli and carrot.

In a food processor, combine the arugula, garlic, and salt and process to a paste. Scrape down and add the olive oil, then process again until smooth. Add the ricotta and Parmesan and process again.

Cook the pasta according to the package directions, and during the last 2 minutes of cooking time, add the broccoli and carrot. Drain well, then return the pasta and veggies to the pot and toss with the pesto and chopped tomato. If desired, stir constantly over medium heat to warm through. Serve warm.

Keeps for 4 days, tightly covered, in the refrigerator.

WHOLE WHEAT PENNE
IN ROASTED-PEPPER ROMESCO SAUCE

Keep a couple jars of roasted red peppers in your pantry, and you will always be ready to make this delicious pasta. Sweet peppers, nuts, and olive oil combine for a taste of Spain, and a nice break from the usual tomato-based pasta sauce. Whole wheat penne carries the sauce to perfection and is just as good the second day, warmed up for lunch.

SERVES 6 (MAKES ABOUT 8 CUPS)

1 medium dried ancho pepper

1 (7½-ounce) jar roasted red peppers, or 1 large (or 2 very small) fresh red bell peppers

½ cup slivered almonds

1 garlic clove

½ teaspoon smoked paprika

½ teaspoon salt

3 tablespoons extra-virgin olive oil

1 tablespoon red wine vinegar

8 ounces whole wheat penne

1 cup peas

½ cup fresh parsley leaves or fresh basil leaves, chopped

Put on a large pot of salted water to boil for the pasta.

Place the ancho pepper in a heat-safe cup and pour boiling water over it to rehydrate. Let stand until soft and pliable, about 30 minutes. Drain the softened pepper and pat dry, then use a paring knife to slice down one side. Open the pepper, remove the stem and seeds, and tear the pepper into chunks.

If using jarred roasted peppers, drain them, rinse, and pat dry. If using fresh, see the directions below.

Toast the almonds in a 350°F oven on a sheet pan, stirring every 5 minutes until golden, for a total of 10 to 15 minutes.

In a food processor or blender, process the almonds to a fine mince. Add the rehydrated ancho pepper, roasted peppers, garlic, paprika, and salt and purée until smooth, stopping to scrape down as necessary. With the machine running, slowly pour in the olive oil and then the vinegar.

Cook the pasta according to the package directions, adding the peas in the last 2 minutes of cooking. Drain well and toss with the sauce in the cooking pot. Stir over low heat to warm through, then stir in the fresh parsley. Serve warm. (This pasta can also be served cold.)

Keeps for 4 days, tightly covered, in the refrigerator.

To prepare freshly roasted peppers, use one large or two very small red bell peppers. To roast the peppers, heat a broiler to high. Put the peppers on a pan 3 inches from the heat and broil until black and blistered on each side, about 4 minutes per side. When all sides are blackened, put the peppers in an airtight, heat-safe container with a lid. A covered casserole dish works well. Let stand for 15 minutes to steam, then remove the lid to cool. When cool enough to handle, peel and seed the peppers and chop coarsely. Proceed with the recipe.

WHOLE WHEAT SPAGHETTI WITH GARLICKY BREADCRUMBS, KALE, AND PARMESAN

Simple pastas like this are the backbone of Italian home cooking. Here, we use up some stale whole wheat bread in the most delicious way, adding garlic and umami-boosting anchovies for an adventure in crunch. Vegetarians can skip the anchovies—just add a pinch more salt. Tuscan kale is the sweetest kale, but you can use any variety, or even substitute Swiss chard or spinach in this delightful dish.

SERVES 4 (MAKES ABOUT 6 CUPS)

2 tablespoons extra-virgin olive oil,
  plus more as desired

2 anchovies, chopped,
  or 1 tablespoon anchovy paste (optional)

6 garlic cloves, minced

¼ teaspoon red pepper flakes

1 cup whole wheat breadcrumbs
  (1 or 2 slices of bread, ground in a food processor)

½ teaspoon salt (or more if you are not using anchovies)

1 bunch (8 ounces) kale (preferably Tuscan),
  stemmed and thinly sliced

8 ounces whole wheat spaghetti

½ cup finely shredded Parmesan cheese

Bring a large pot of salted water to a boil for the pasta. In a large skillet over medium-high heat, warm the oil. Add the anchovies (if using), garlic, and red pepper flakes and cook until fragrant, about 1 minute. Stir in the breadcrumbs and cook until golden, 2 to 3 minutes. Add the salt and kale and stir until the kale is wilted, about 2 minutes. Take off the heat while you cook the pasta.

Cook the spaghetti according to the package directions and drain well. Toss in the sauté pan with the crumb mixture until all the pasta is coated and well mixed, then add the Parmesan and toss again. Serve hot.

Keeps for 4 days, tightly covered, in the refrigerator.

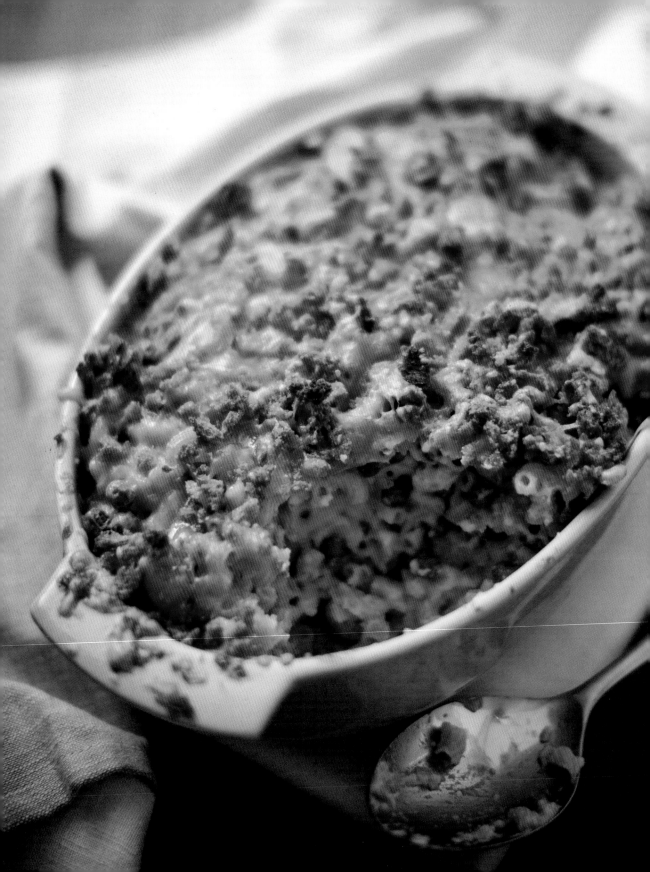

WHOLE GRAIN MAC *AND* CHEESE WITH PEAS

Go ahead, serve your family these crunchy, crumb-topped creamy noodles and watch them dig in. You don't have to tell them that there are hidden sweet potatoes and onions puréed into the cheesy sauce, adding to the vegetable content of the meal, or that the macaroni is made from healthy whole grain. Why say anything? Just listen to the happy sounds of people enjoying a cheesy mac.

SERVES 6 (MAKES 8 CUPS)

1 tablespoon canola oil, plus more for the pan

2 cups (8 ounces) chopped sweet potato

1 cup chopped onion

2 cups milk

1/8 teaspoon ground nutmeg

1 teaspoon salt

8 ounces sharp Cheddar cheese, shredded (3 cups), divided

4 ounces Gruyère, shredded (1½ cups), divided

½ teaspoon cider vinegar

12 ounces whole wheat macaroni

1 cup frozen peas

2 slices whole wheat bread (1½ cups breadcrumbs)

2 teaspoons unsalted butter or olive oil

Preheat the oven to 400°F. Lightly oil a 2-quart baking dish. Put on a large pot of salted water to boil for the macaroni.

In a large sauté pan, heat the canola oil over medium heat and sauté the sweet potatoes and onion. Turn the heat to low and cover the pan, cooking for about 5 minutes, or until the sweet potatoes are very soft when pierced with a paring knife. Transfer the sweet potatoes and onion to a food processor and purée until smooth, scraping down as necessary.

Pour the milk into the sauté pan and warm it over medium heat just until hot to the touch (don't boil). Transfer the hot milk to the processor and add the nutmeg, salt, 2 cups of the Cheddar, 1/2 cup of the Gruyère, and the cider vinegar. Process until smooth. The cheese should melt from being mixed with the hot milk and vegetables.

Cook the macaroni for 2 minutes less than the package instructs (it should be a little underdone). Put the peas in the colander and drain the hot macaroni over the peas. Shake the colander to dry the pasta and peas. Transfer into the prepared 2-quart baking dish and pour the cheese sauce over, stirring to mix. Make the breadcrumbs by tearing the bread into coarse pieces, then pulsing into large crumbs in the food processor. In a medium bowl, combine the remaining cheeses, breadcrumbs, and butter or oil. Sprinkle evenly over the top of the macaroni.

Bake for about 30 minutes, or until bubbly and browned on top.

Once cooled, keeps for 1 week, tightly covered, in the refrigerator.

SAVORY SPINACH *AND* CHEESE BREAD PUDDING

Bread puddings aren't just for dessert. In this lovely casserole, whole wheat bread soaks up custardy eggs and becomes a completely new food. Dappled with spinach and sprinkled with Parmesan, it's a whole grain egg bake for any meal of the day.

SERVES 8

1 tablespoon extra-virgin olive oil, plus more for the pan

1 (8-ounce) package button mushrooms, chopped

1 large onion, chopped

8 ounces fresh spinach, coarsely chopped

8 cups cubed whole wheat bread

1½ cups milk

6 large eggs

4 ounces Parmesan cheese, shredded, divided

½ teaspoon salt

½ teaspoon freshly ground black pepper

1 tablespoon fresh marjoram

Preheat the oven to 375°F. Lightly oil a 2-quart baking dish. In a large sauté pan, heat the olive oil, then add the mushrooms and onion and sauté over medium-high heat for about 5 minutes, or until the mushrooms are browned and the pan is dry. Add the spinach and stir, then take off the heat and continue to stir until the spinach is wilted. Add the bread cubes if your pan is large enough, or you can add them to the mix in the next step. In a large bowl, whisk together the milk, egg, and half of the Parmesan cheese, then stir in the salt, pepper, and marjoram. Add the mushroom mixture and bread cubes and fold in gently.

Transfer to the prepared pan and press flat with a spatula. Top with the remaining Parmesan. Bake for 45 minutes, or until the middle is puffed and the cheese is browned. Insert a paring knife into the center of the pan, and if it comes out with no raw egg on it, it is done. Cool for 5 minutes or so before serving.

Once cooled, keeps for 1 week, tightly covered, in the refrigerator.

WHOLE GRAIN SOUR CREAM _with_ DILL NOODLES

These quick and creamy noodles are a perfect side to a simple roasted salmon fillet or a Swedish meatball. Just a bit of sour cream goes a long way in the stock-enhanced sauce, so they are not too decadent.

SERVES 3 (MAKES 3½ CUPS)
1 tablespoon unsalted butter
1 tablespoon unbleached flour
½ cup chicken or vegetable stock
¼ cup sour cream
2 tablespoons fresh dill leaves, finely chopped
½ teaspoon salt
½ cup frozen peas, thawed
8 ounces whole wheat egg noodles

Put on a large pot of salted water to boil for the noodles. In a 4-quart saucepan, melt the butter, then whisk in the flour. Cook for a couple of minutes, or until bubbly. Take off the heat and gradually whisk in the stock until smooth. Stir in the sour cream, dill, and salt and keep warm.

Put the peas in the colander that you will use to drain the noodles. Cook the noodles according to the package directions and pour the pasta and water over the peas in the colander. Drain well. Stir the noodles and peas into the sour cream sauce and serve warm.

Once cooled, keeps for 4 days, tightly covered, in the refrigerator.

SAVORY KASHA *with* PARSNIPS

Kasha is toasted buckwheat, and it tastes nutty and earthy. Add sweet parsnips and you have a real celebration of intense plant flavors. Pair this with herbed roasted meats, or add a handful of toasted walnuts for a vegetarian meal.

SERVES 4 (MAKES 4 CUPS)

1 tablespoon extra-virgin olive oil
1 medium onion, chopped
5 ounces parsnip, chopped (1 cup)
1 cup buckwheat groats
1 sprig fresh rosemary
½ teaspoon salt
½ teaspoon freshly ground black pepper
1½ cups vegetable or chicken stock
½ cup chopped fresh parsley

In a 4-quart pot, heat the oil briefly over medium-high heat and add the onion and parsnip. Stir for 5 to 10 minutes, or until the onion is golden and soft. Add the buckwheat and stir for a couple of minutes. Add the rosemary, salt, and pepper and stir, then add the stock and bring to a boil. Cover and reduce the heat to the lowest setting. Cook for 15 minutes, or until the liquids are all absorbed, then let stand for 5 minutes, covered, off the heat.

Fluff the hot grain and fold in the parsley. Serve warm.

Once cooled, keeps for 1 week, tightly covered, in the refrigerator.

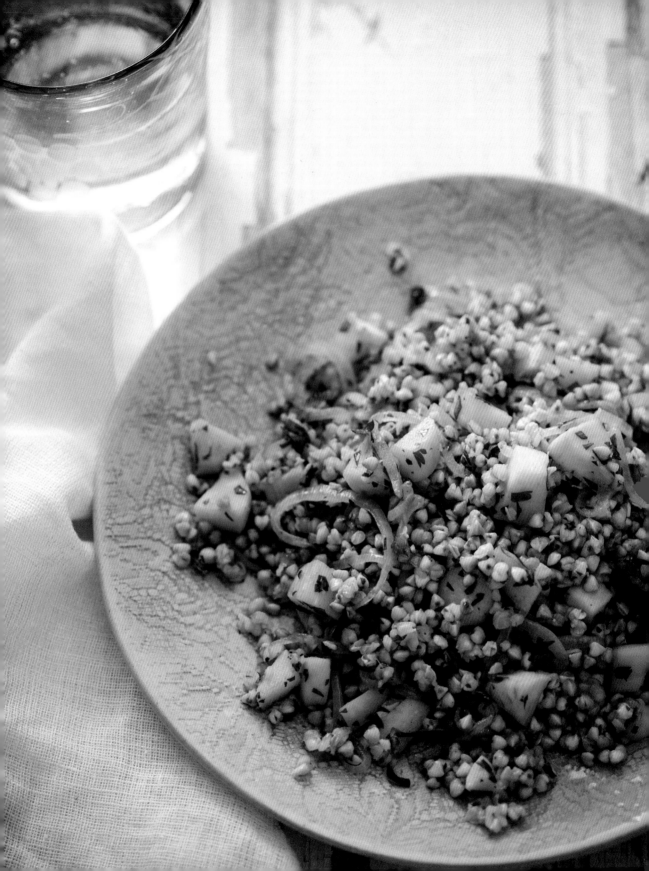

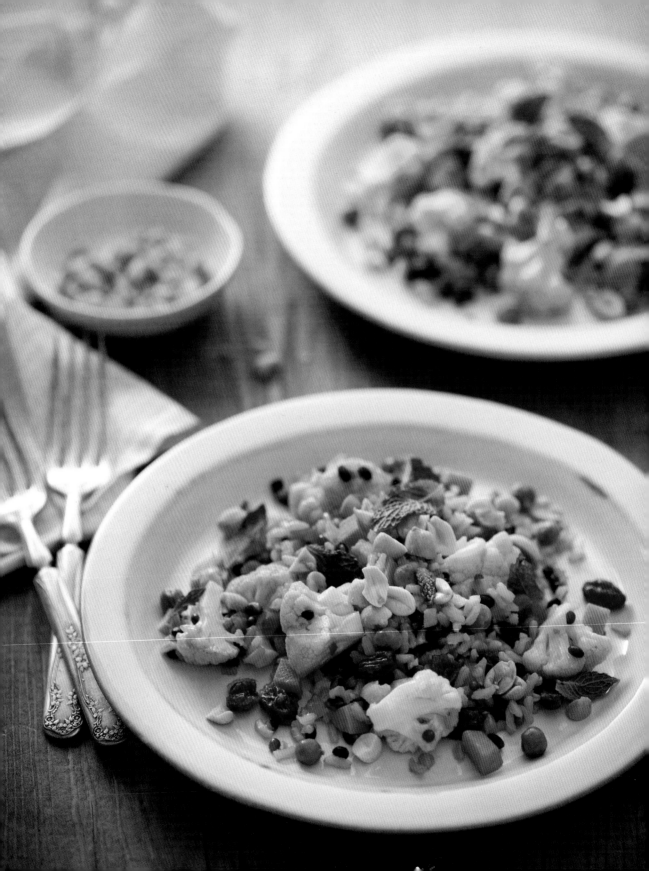

INDIAN YELLOW MIXED-GRAIN BIRYANI

In a traditional Indian meal, yellow rice anchors the plate, and all sorts of little dishes provide a variety of sweet, sour, and spicy flavors to alternate between. In this dish, veggies cook with the tinted rice, making a whole grain– and vegetable-rich side. This is a delicious counterpoint to dal soups, spinach dishes, and curries of all sorts, especially served with chutney on the side.

SERVES 4 (MAKES 4 CUPS)

1 tablespoon canola oil

1 medium red onion, chopped

1 tablespoon chopped fresh ginger

1 teaspoon turmeric

3 garlic cloves, chopped

½ teaspoon red pepper flakes (optional)

1 teaspoon cumin seeds

1 teaspoon brown mustard seeds

1 stick cinnamon

1 bay leaf

2 cups water

1 cup brown rice blend

½ teaspoon salt

1½ cups (6 ounces) cauliflower florets

1 large carrot, chopped

½ cup frozen peas, thawed

½ cup raisins or dried currants

½ cup fresh mint leaves

½ cup roasted peanuts, chopped

In a 6-quart pan, heat the canola oil and sauté the red onion over medium-high heat. When the onion is soft, add the ginger, turmeric, garlic, red pepper flakes, cumin seeds, mustard seeds, cinnamon stick, and bay leaf. Cook, stirring, until the spices are fragrant. Add the water, rice, and salt and bring to a boil, then reduce the heat to low and cover. Cook for 30 minutes.

Uncover, stir, and add the cauliflower, carrot, and peas. Cover and cook for 10 minutes more. Uncover and test the rice; it should be tender. Let stand, covered, for 5 minutes to finish steaming the grain. Serve topped with raisins, mint, and peanuts.

Once cooled, keeps for 1 week, tightly covered, in the refrigerator.

VEGGIE *AND* BROWN RICE MEDLEY

In this recipe, you will find a template. You see, when you cook brown rice, or any long-cooking grain, you can always add some vegetables to the pot so that they get cooked, too. The brown rice, cabbage, and rosemary in this dish can easily be subbed with black rice, bok choy, and ginger, or wheat berries, turnips, and thyme.

SERVES 4 (MAKES 4 CUPS)

1 teaspoon extra-virgin olive oil
1 small onion, chopped
1 stalk celery, chopped
1 medium carrot, chopped
2 cups chopped cabbage or kale
2 sprigs fresh rosemary
½ teaspoon salt
½ teaspoon freshly ground black pepper
1 cup long-grain brown rice
1½ cups vegetable or chicken stock
Sliced almonds, toasted (optional)

In a 4-quart pot, heat the olive oil for a few seconds over medium-high heat, then add the onion, celery, carrot, and cabbage or kale. Stir for 5 minutes, or until the onion is soft and golden. Add the fresh rosemary and stir, then add the salt, pepper, brown rice, and stock. Turn the heat to high. When the stock comes to a boil, reduce the heat to low and cover the pot tightly.

Cook for 40 to 45 minutes. When all the liquids are absorbed and the rice is tender, take the pot off the heat. Let stand for 5 minutes to finish steaming. Serve topped with almonds, if desired.

Once cooled, keeps for 1 week, tightly covered, in the refrigerator.

ANY-GRAIN FRIED "RICE" *with* VEGGIES AND EGG

Chinese fried rice is the ultimate repurposing of a leftover. Why not make the same magic with leftover whole grains? That pot of grain that you cooked at the beginning of the week can transform into a fast and satisfying weeknight meal, with some veggies and an egg thrown in.

SERVES 5 (MAKES ABOUT 5 CUPS)

3 cups cooked grain (about 1 cup uncooked)

1 tablespoon chopped fresh ginger

2 garlic cloves, chopped

3 tablespoons soy sauce

2 tablespoons packed light brown sugar
  or other sweetener

1 teaspoon toasted sesame oil

2 large eggs

1 tablespoon canola oil

1½ cups (4 ounces) snow peas, trimmed

4 large scallions, chopped into 1-inch pieces
  (white and green parts)

1 (5-ounce) can sliced water chestnuts, drained

Let the grain come to room temperature if it is cold, and break up any lumps with your fingers. In a cup, stir together the ginger, garlic, soy sauce, brown sugar, and sesame oil. In another cup, whisk the eggs and reserve.

In a wok or large skillet, heat the canola oil over high heat until hot, swirling to coat the pan. Add the snow peas, scallions, water chestnuts, and cooked grain, stirring over medium-high heat until the peas are crisp-tender. Stir the soy sauce mixture again to recombine and pour over the grain and veggies in the pan, stirring to mix.

Pour the eggs into the hot pan, stirring to coat the grain. Keep stirring until the eggs are cooked; the mixture will look dry and less shiny. Serve hot.

Once cooled, keeps for 1 week, tightly covered, in the refrigerator.

BARLEY *AND* SWEET POTATO TIMBALES

Take advantage of the slightly sticky texture of cooked barley and mold the cooked grain in a cup, then tap out on a plate. This chewy, sweet potato–studded dish would be delicious in any form, but the visual appeal of a shaped portion exponentially increases the enjoyment.

SERVES 4

2 teaspoons unsalted butter

¼ cup diced onion

½ cup chopped sweet potato

1 cup pearled barley

2½ cups chicken or vegetable stock

½ teaspoon ground cumin

½ teaspoon salt

Canola oil, for the ramekins

½ cup shredded Parmesan cheese

1 cup fresh spinach leaves, shredded

In a small saucepan with a tight-fitting lid, melt the butter and then add the onion and sweet potato. Sauté over medium heat until the onion is soft, about 5 minutes. Add the barley and stir until heated through, then add the stock, cumin, and salt. Bring to a boil, reduce to a simmer, then cover tightly and cook for 30 minutes. Lightly oil four 1-cup ramekins.

When all the liquid is absorbed, take off the heat and let stand, covered, for 5 minutes. Stir the Parmesan into the hot barley. Scoop the barley into the ramekins and pack it in well. At this point, the timbales can hold in a warm oven for 1 hour until serving.

To serve, invert each ramekin over a small plate and tap to release the grain. Garnish with shredded spinach leaves and serve immediately.

Once cooled, keeps for 1 week, tightly covered, in the refrigerator.

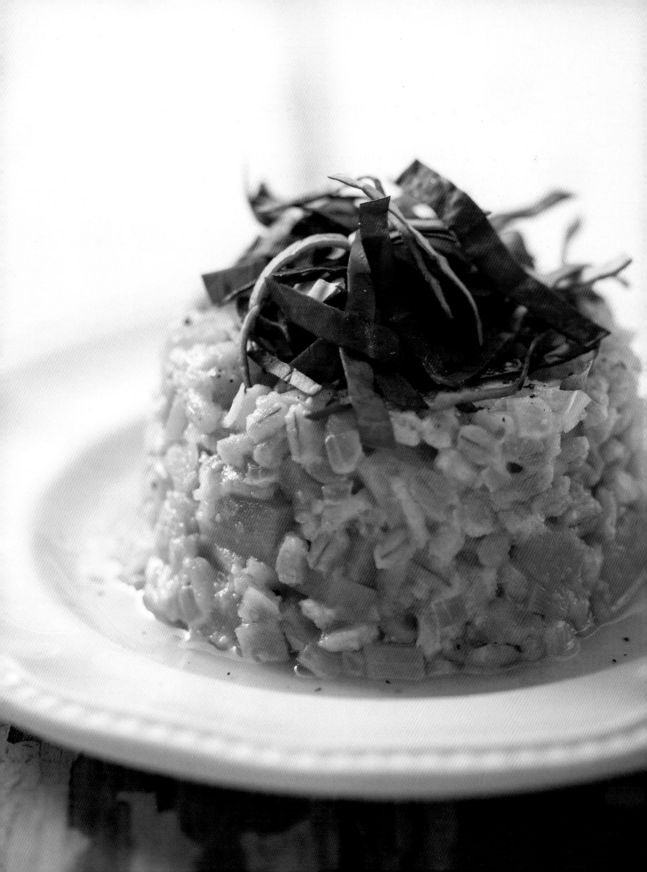

QUINOA *AND* SUN-DRIED TOMATO TIMBALES

These delicate, flavor-splashed timbales can serve as a filling side dish or a lovely vegetarian main course. Intensely flavored dried tomatoes and creamy, salty feta complement the subtle grassiness of quinoa in a delightful way. Make extra—these pack well for lunch or snacks.

SERVES 4

Canola oil, for the ramekins
1 teaspoon canola oil
½ cup chopped onion
¾ cup quinoa
½ teaspoon salt
1½ cups chicken or vegetable stock
½ cup sun-dried tomato halves, rehydrated and chopped
1 teaspoon dried basil
2 large eggs, lightly whisked
4 large scallions, chopped, divided (white and green parts)
4 ounces feta cheese, cubed

Oil four 1-cup ramekins for the timbales and reserve.

In a 2-quart saucepan, heat the canola oil and sauté the onion until soft and translucent and beginning to brown. Add the quinoa and stir to coat, then add the salt and stock and bring to a boil. Cover and reduce the heat to the lowest setting. Cook for about 15 minutes, or until all the liquid is absorbed. Transfer the cooked quinoa to a large bowl and cool to room temperature. Stir in the sun-dried tomatoes and basil.

Preheat the oven to 400°F. Set the prepared ramekins on a sheet pan. To the quinoa, add the eggs and stir to mix. Stir in half the scallions and all of the feta, and divide between the ramekins. Bake for 20 minutes, or until puffed and set.

Let cool on a rack for about 5 minutes before running a paring knife around the edges and inverting onto small plates. Garnish with the remaining scallions and serve.

Once cooled, keeps for 1 week, tightly covered, in the refrigerator.

POTATO-GRAIN CROQUETTES
WITH WARM HONEY-MUSTARD SAUCE

When you want some crispy, kid-friendly food, make these croquettes. Bound by soft potato mash, the whole grains make a chewy, hearty base for a handful of herbs. Everyone loves a croquette with a tasty sauce, and as long as they are whole grain, it's a win-win!

SERVES 6 (MAKES ABOUT 24 CAKES)

Canola oil, for the pan

2½ cups cooked short-grain brown rice, quinoa, millet,
   or buckwheat groats (a little less than 1 cup uncooked)

2 large Yukon gold potatoes (11 ounces)

¼ cup chopped fresh parsley

2 tablespoons fresh dill leaves, chopped

1 teaspoon salt

1 large egg

¼ cup Dijon mustard

¼ cup honey

½ teaspoon freshly ground black pepper

Pinch of salt

Oil a large sheet pan and reserve.

Preheat the oven to 400°F.

Cook the grain, or if using leftover cooked grain, let it come to room temperature. Boil the potatoes whole until tender and easily pierced with a paring knife, then drain. When cool enough to handle, slip off the skins and mash the potato, then let cool. When the grain and potatoes are at room temperature, combine them in a large bowl and add the parsley, dill, salt, and egg and mix well to make a thick mash.

Scoop 2-tablespoon-sized portions and form into flattened disks about ¾ inch thick. Place on the sheet pan with a little room between them (they will not spread).

Bake for 15 minutes, then take out the pan and flip the croquettes over with a metal spatula. Return to the oven and bake for 10 minutes more. They will be golden brown on the top and bottom.

While the croquettes bake, stir together the mustard, honey, pepper, and salt.

To warm the sauce, heat gently in a pan or in the microwave. Serve the croquettes hot, with the honey-mustard sauce on the side.

Once cooled, the croquettes and sauce keep for 1 week, tightly covered, in the refrigerator.

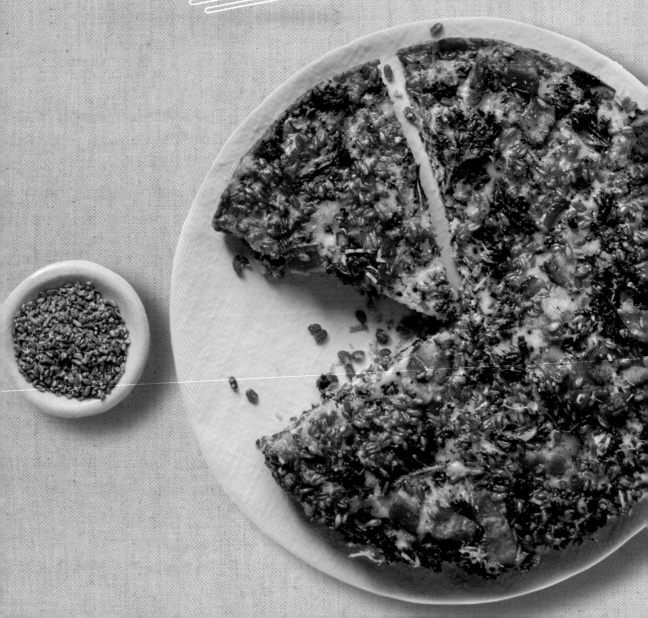

MAIN COURSES

EASY BLACK BEAN BURGERS WITH OATS *AND* AVOCADO SALSA

Take a break from beef and try this tasty veggie burger packed with all kinds of flavors and textures. Tender beans and chewy oats provide plenty of excitement, and once you add the creamy avocado salsa, you'll forget about the old burgers.

SERVES 4

SALSA

1 small avocado, diced

½ cup chopped tomato

1 small jalapeño pepper, minced

2 teaspoons freshly squeezed lime juice

¼ teaspoon salt

BURGERS

1 (15-ounce) can black beans, drained and rinsed, divided

1 cup rolled oats

2 large eggs

1 teaspoon salt

1½ teaspoons ground cumin

½ teaspoon ground chipotle pepper, or more to taste

1 large scallion, minced (white and green parts)

2 tablespoons chopped fresh cilantro

2 ounces sharp Cheddar cheese, finely shredded (½ cup)

Canola oil, for the pan

4 whole wheat hamburger buns

First, make the salsa. Combine the avocado, tomato, jalapeño, lime, and salt in a medium bowl and toss to mix. Cover and keep cool while you make the burgers.

For the burgers, transfer half of the beans to a large bowl. Put the oats in a food processor and pulse three times, or until chopped. Add the other half of the beans to the processor and pulse to a coarse paste. Add the eggs, salt, cumin, and chipotle and process to mix well, about 1 minute. Add the contents of the processor to the bowl with the remaining beans and stir in the scallion, cilantro, and cheese. Spray a plate with vegetable oil spray. Using wet hands, divide the bean mixture into four portions of about ½ cup each, form into patties about ¾ inch thick, and place them on the prepared plate. Chill for 10 to 15 minutes.

Preheat a large skillet or cast-iron pan on high heat for a minute, then brush or spray with oil. The pan should be very hot. Fry the burgers for 2 to 3 minutes on the first side to brown and form a good crust, then carefully flip to the other side. Cook for another 3 to 5 minutes, flipping if necessary, until the burgers feel firm when pressed. Toast the buns, if desired, then serve with the avocado salsa spooned on the burgers.

Once cooked, the burgers keep for 4 days, tightly covered, in the refrigerator.

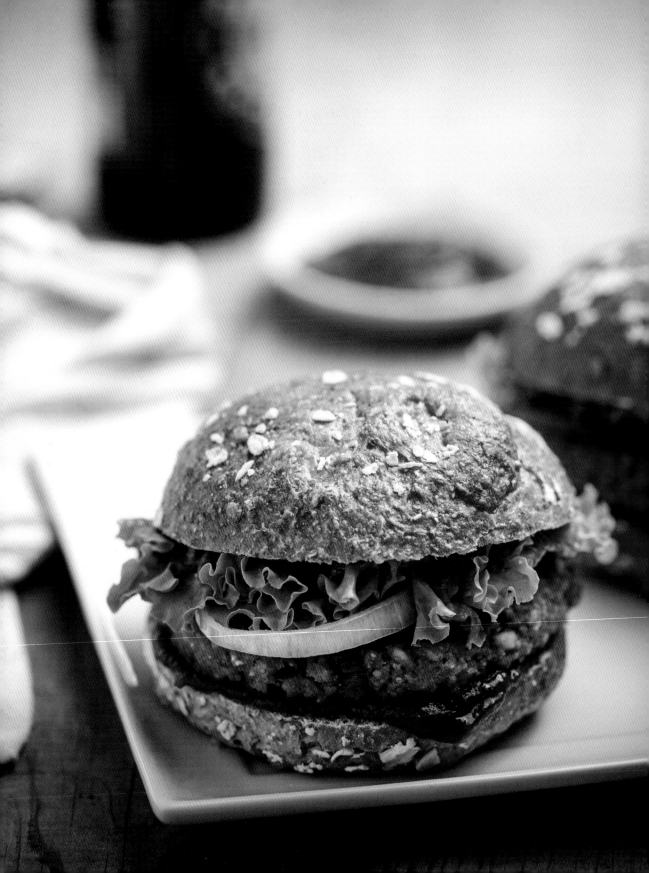

PECAN AND BARLEY BURGERS *WITH* PEACH KETCHUP

Bake up a batch of these chewy, nutty burgers and then slather them with the tangy peach ketchup for a taste of summer. This recipe makes eight burgers, so if you have any left over, note that they keep well to pack for lunch or dinner and are equally good in a lettuce leaf with a drizzle of Sriracha.

BURGERS

SERVES 8

Canola oil, for the pan

2 cups water

1 cup barley, red rice, or buckwheat groats

1 cup pecan halves

1½ cups sweet potato purée
(1 large sweet potato, baked, peeled, and coarsely mashed)

¼ cup ground flax seeds

1 tablespoon Dijon mustard

2 tablespoons whole wheat flour

1 teaspoon salt

½ teaspoon freshly ground black pepper

1 teaspoon ground cumin

1 teaspoon ground coriander

4 medium scallions, chopped
(white and green parts)

8 whole wheat buns or lettuce leaves
(for lettuce wraps)

KETCHUP

SERVES 8 (MAKES 1½ CUPS)

2 large peaches, peeled and chopped (2 cups)

2 tablespoons maple syrup

1 teaspoon molasses

1 tablespoon cider vinegar

½ teaspoon paprika

¼ teaspoon garlic powder

¼ teaspoon salt

Pinch of cinnamon

Bring the water to a boil in a pot and add the barley. Cook until tender, about 40 minutes. Drain and let cool.

Preheat the oven to 400°F. Oil a sheet pan and reserve.

In a food processor, pulse the pecans until finely chopped. Add 2 cups of the cooked barley to the processor and pulse to make a coarse purée. Add the sweet potato, flax, Dijon, flour, salt, pepper, cumin, coriander, and scallions and process to mix. Scrape into a bowl and stir in the remaining cooked barley.

Use a ½-cup measure to scoop the mixture onto the oiled pan, leaving space between portions. Oil your palms and flatten the portions into ¾-inch-thick burgers.

Bake for 20 minutes, then use a spatula to flip the burgers. Bake for another 20 minutes, or until firm when pressed with your finger. Cool in the pan on a rack or serve hot.

Make the ketchup. In a small pot, combine the peaches, maple syrup, molasses, vinegar, paprika, garlic powder, salt, and cinnamon. Bring to a boil over medium-high heat, then reduce the heat and simmer vigorously for about 10 minutes. Mash the peaches coarsely with a fork to thicken, or purée for a smoother sauce. Cool completely.

Serve the burgers on buns or in individual lettuce leaves, with ketchup to taste. The burgers keep for 1 week, tightly covered, in the refrigerator.

QUINOA-FETA PHYLLO TRIANGLES

We have all had rich, buttery spanakopita. In this lightened-up version, a little feta graces the crave-worthy quinoa-spinach center, and the crispy phyllo is brushed with healthy olive oil. The filling is so good, in fact, that you could just skip the wrapper and eat it as is.

SERVES 8 (MAKES 8 TRIANGLES)

1 pound fresh spinach

¼ cup plus 1 tablespoon extra-virgin olive oil, divided

1 medium onion, chopped

1 (2-inch) sliver of pared lemon zest, left whole

½ cup quinoa

¾ cup water

¼ teaspoon salt

1 teaspoon dried oregano

½ teaspoon freshly ground black pepper

1 large egg

¼ cup dried currants

4 ounces feta cheese, rinsed and crumbled

½ pound phyllo dough (8 whole sheets), thawed

Bring a large pot of water to a boil, drop in the spinach, and stir for 1 minute, or until the leaves are wilted. Drain and rinse with cold water. When the leaves are wilted, drain and rinse with cold water. Let cool, then wring out the spinach and roll up in a kitchen towel to dry completely.

In a 1-quart pot, heat 1 tablespoon of the olive oil over medium heat and add the onion. Sauté, stirring frequently, for about 10 minutes. Add the lemon zest, quinoa, water, and salt and raise the heat to bring it to a boil. Once boiling, cover tightly and reduce the heat to low. Cook for 15 minutes, or until all the water is absorbed. Let cool to room temperature. Remove the lemon zest.

Preheat the oven to 400°F. Line a sheet pan with parchment paper. In a large bowl, combine the oregano, pepper, and egg and stir to mix. Add the cooked quinoa mixture, spinach, currants, and feta and mix gently. Reserve.

Get out a pastry brush and pour ¼ cup olive oil into a cup.

Unwrap the phyllo and unroll it on a cutting board or counter, then cover with plastic wrap so it won't dry out as you work. Keep a damp towel on top to hold it down flat.

Place a sheet of phyllo on the counter, with the long side closest to you. Dab olive oil over the right half, then fold the left half over to cover it. Dab oil over the right half of the folded piece and fold the left half over again, making a long strip. Place ½ cup of filling on the end of the strip closest to you and fold the bottom right corner up to cover the filling and align the edge with the left edge of the dough. This will form a triangle. Keep folding this way, maintaining a triangular pastry, until you reach the end of the strip. Paint the phyllo triangle lightly with oil and place on the prepared pan. Repeat with the remaining phyllo sheets and filling.

Bake the pies for 15 to 20 minutes, or until the phyllo is crisp and golden. Serve hot.

Once cooled, keeps for 1 week, tightly covered, in the refrigerator.

LIME FISH CAKES WITH BROWN RICE *AND* DIPPING SAUCE

These tangy, crispy-crusted little cakes are a great way to make a piece of fish feed a family. They are also an amazingly appealing appetizer course or a finger food for parties. Black rice gives them a bit of heft, filling you up as you nosh.

SERVES 3 TO 4 (MAKES 12 PIECES)

Canola oil, for the pan and frying

½ cup black rice, red rice, or short-grain brown rice (about 1½ cups cooked)

2 garlic cloves, peeled

1 tablespoon chopped fresh ginger

¾ pound salmon, boned and skinned, chopped into ¾-inch chunks

Freshly grated zest of 1 large lime

4 tablespoons freshly squeezed lime juice, divided

¾ teaspoon salt

¾ teaspoon red pepper flakes, divided

1 large egg

2 medium scallions, chopped (white and green parts)

½ cup sesame seeds

¼ cup fresh cilantro leaves, chopped

2 tablespoons granulated sugar

¼ cup fish sauce

Prepare a sheet pan for the formed fish cakes by lining it with parchment paper and rubbing it lightly with oil. Line a large plate with paper towels to drain the finished cakes.

Cook the rice according to the chart on page 20 and measure out 1½ cups finished rice. Let cool to room temperature.

In a food processor, mince the garlic and ginger. Add the chopped salmon, lime zest, 2 tablespoons of the lime juice, salt, and ¼ teaspoon red pepper flakes. Pulse to chop the salmon coarsely. Add the egg, rice, and scallions and pulse to mix.

Pour the sesame seeds into a wide bowl. Use a #70 scoop or a tablespoon to form 2-tablespoon-sized portions of the fish mixture. Shape each into a round patty and place in the sesame seeds; flatten the patty slightly to about a ¾-inch thickness, lightly coating both sides with seeds. Place on the sheet pan and chill until time to cook.

Make the dipping sauce by combining the remaining 2 tablespoons lime juice, cilantro, ½ teaspoon red pepper flakes, sugar, and fish sauce.

To cook the cakes, place a wide skillet over high heat and pour in canola oil to cover the bottom of the pan. When the oil shimmers, after about 1 minute, carefully place half of the fish cakes in the hot oil. Cook for about 2 minutes on the first side and 1 minute on the second side. Test for doneness by cutting one in half. When cooked through, transfer to the paper towel–lined plate. Repeat with the remaining cakes, adding oil to the pan as needed. Serve hot with the dipping sauce.

Keeps for 3 days, tightly covered, in the refrigerator.

RED QUINOA-CRUSTED BAKED FISH _with_ CUCUMBER-LIME SALSA

Just about any kind of fish is made more exciting by a crispy coating of colorful quinoa. The coating is also packed with protein and hardly any oil—in contrast to your typical battered-fish preparation—so it's a definite step up. The salsa is so quick and charming that you will love making it on a summer night.

SERVES 4

½ cup red quinoa

Canola oil, for the pan

SALSA

1 large cucumber, peeled, seeded, and chopped

1 cup cubed fresh pineapple (about ¼ small pineapple)

1 large jalapeño pepper, seeded and chopped

½ cup fresh cilantro leaves, chopped

1 tablespoon freshly squeezed lime juice

½ teaspoon salt

FISH

2 tablespoons white whole wheat flour

1 teaspoon salt

2 large eggs

1½ pounds firm white fish fillets, such as perch, cod, or haddock

Bring a pot of water to a boil and drop in the quinoa for 10 minutes, then drain well in a fine-mesh strainer. Spread the quinoa on a kitchen towel to dry. Transfer from the damp towel to a sheet pan and let air-dry until it no longer feels wet to the touch. Transfer to a medium bowl.

Preheat the oven to 425°F. Lightly oil a sheet pan or an oven-safe dish large enough to hold all the fish in a single layer.

Make the salsa: Combine the cucumber, pineapple, jalapeño, cilantro, lime juice, and salt in a bowl and stir.

For the fish: Put the flour in a medium bowl and stir in the salt. Whisk the eggs in another bowl. Toss the fish fillets in the flour mixture to coat. Dip each in egg, then coat with quinoa and place it on the baking sheet or pan, making sure the fillets do not touch.

Bake for 15 minutes for ¾-inch-thick fillets, or up to 20 minutes for thicker fillets like cod. Serve hot with the salsa on the side.

These are best served hot and fresh but will keep 3 days, tightly covered, in the refrigerator.

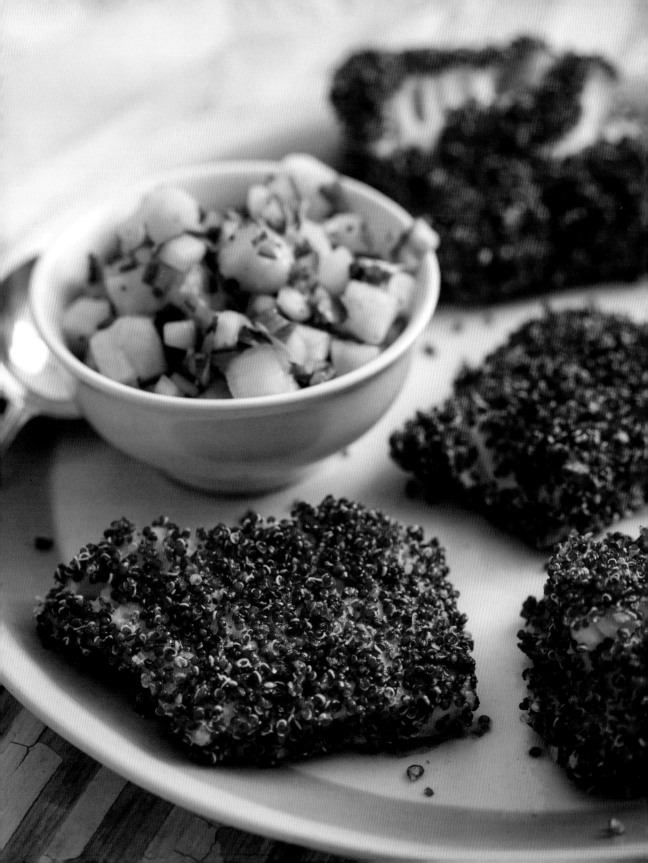

BAKED SOLE FILLED WITH LEMONY DILL PILAF

Delicate sole fillets stay moist and delicious in this easy, baked dish. A strip of lemon zest infuses the rice, and there is just enough cheese to make it creamy. Cradling an herb-infused filling, the fish is shown off to great effect—now all you need is a salad for a complete meal.

SERVES 4

1 teaspoon extra-virgin olive oil, plus more for the pan

1 large scallion, chopped (white and green parts)

1 medium carrot, finely chopped

1 cup long-grain brown rice

1³/₄ cups vegetable or chicken stock

¹/₂ teaspoon salt

1 (3-inch) sliver of pared lemon zest, left whole

1 teaspoon freshly squeezed lemon juice

2 ounces chèvre cheese or cream cheese

2 tablespoons fresh dill leaves, chopped, plus sprigs for garnish

1 (2-pound) sole fillet, cut into 8 pieces

¹/₂ teaspoon paprika

Lemon wedges, for serving

Lightly oil a 1-quart baking dish with a lid or an 8-inch square baking pan that you can cover with foil. In a 1-quart pot, heat the olive oil for a few seconds, then add the scallion and carrot. Stir over medium-high heat until the scallion is softened, about 2 minutes. Add the brown rice, stock, salt, and lemon zest strip and bring to a boil. Cover tightly, reduce the heat to low, and cook for 35 to 40 minutes. When the rice is tender and all the liquids have been absorbed, take off the heat and let cool, covered, for 5 minutes. Fold in the lemon juice, chèvre, and dill. Remove the lemon zest. Let cool to room temperature.

Preheat the oven to 375°F.

Place a layer of paper towels on the cutting board and pat dry the sole, if necessary. If the pieces are thicker than ¹/₄ inch, carefully halve them lengthwise into wide, long strips. Lay all the sole on the board and portion the cooked rice mixture to cover three fourths of each piece of fish. (There will be filling left over for the next step.) Roll them up like cinnamon rolls, starting with the covered part. Secure each with a toothpick and keep on the board. Sprinkle with paprika.

In the prepared baking pan, spread the leftover rice mixture loosely across the bottom. Place the fish rolls on top, nestling them into the rice so that they stay upright. Cover and bake for 20 minutes, or until the fish will flake easily. Garnish with dill sprigs and lemon wedges and serve.

Once cooled, keeps for 3 days, tightly covered, in the refrigerator.

GRAIN AND NUT BALLS
WITH MARINARA AND WHOLE WHEAT PENNE

These meatless "meatballs" take full advantage of the meaty qualities of chewy whole grains and the satisfying heft of walnuts. Add all the Italian flavors of herbs, tomatoes, and pasta, and you have a new classic for Meatless Mondays.

SERVES 8 (MAKES ABOUT 40)

2 tablespoons extra-virgin olive oil, plus more for the pan

2 large onions, chopped, divided

4 garlic cloves, chopped

1 cup walnuts, lightly toasted

2 cups cooked brown rice, buckwheat groats, or millet

1 teaspoon dried thyme

1 teaspoon dried basil

2 teaspoons dried oregano, divided

1 teaspoon dried sage

1 teaspoon salt, divided

3 tablespoons whole wheat pastry flour

1/2 cup shredded carrot

1 (14 1/2-ounce) can diced tomatoes, with juice

1/4 cup tomato paste

1/2 cup red wine

1/4 cup fresh parsley leaves, chopped

12 ounces whole wheat penne

1/2 cup fresh basil leaves, shredded, for garnish (optional)

Preheat the oven to 400°F. Prepare a sheet pan by lining it with parchment paper and lightly oiling it. In a large skillet over medium heat, warm the oil. Add the onions and garlic and sauté until the onions are golden, about 10 minutes, then transfer half of the mixture to a 4-quart pot to make the sauce. In a food processor, coarsely chop the walnuts. Add the remaining onions from the pan, the cooked grain, 1 teaspoon each thyme, basil, oregano, and sage, 1/2 teaspoon of the salt, and the pastry flour and pulse to combine and mix well.

Lightly oil a #70 scoop or a tablespoon and scoop 2-tablespoon-sized portions and form into "meatballs." Place on the prepared pan, not touching. Bake for 15 minutes, then flip the balls and bake for 15 minutes more. Keep warm until time to serve.

While the balls bake, make the sauce. Heat the reserved sautéed onions in the 4-quart pot and add the carrot. Sauté until the carrot is slightly softened, about 3 minutes. Add the diced tomatoes and bring to a boil. In a cup, stir together the tomato paste and wine and then stir that into the tomatoes in the pan. Add the remaining teaspoon oregano, parsley, and remaining 1/2 teaspoon salt and bring to a boil, then reduce to just a simmer. Cook on low heat until the sauce is thickened.

When the "meatballs" are done, cook the pasta according to the package directions, about 10 minutes, then drain well. In the pasta pot, combine the sauce, pasta, and "meatballs" and stir gently. Heat on medium to warm all the elements, then serve topped with fresh basil, if desired.

Keeps for 5 days, tightly covered, in the refrigerator.

PESTO TURKEY LOAF ᵂᴵᵀᴴ OATS

If you have ever wanted to cut back on meat but not give it up entirely, this is the recipe for you. Stretch a pound of lean ground turkey by adding oats that are plumped with chicken or beef stock, and you have a real winner. A stripe of herby pesto and a topping of tangy tomato sauce give it plenty of flavor for the whole family to enjoy.

SERVES 8

2 large eggs

1 cup rolled oats

¾ cup beef stock

1 medium onion, chopped

½ teaspoon salt

½ teaspoon freshly ground black pepper

1 pound ground turkey

1 garlic clove, peeled

2 tablespoons pine nuts or walnuts

1 cup fresh basil leaves

1 tablespoon extra-virgin olive oil,
  plus more for the pan

TOPPING

½ cup tomato paste

3 tablespoons balsamic vinegar

1 tablespoon packed light brown sugar

Preheat the oven to 350°F. Lightly oil or spray an 8 x 3⁷/₈ x 2¹/₂-inch loaf pan. In a large bowl, combine the eggs, oats, stock, onion, salt, and pepper and mix well. Add the ground turkey and mix well.

In a food processor, combine the garlic, nuts, and basil and process until finely ground. Add the olive oil, scrape down, and purée until well combined.

Transfer half of the turkey mixture to the prepared loaf pan and smooth the top. Sprinkle the pesto mixture evenly over the turkey and then dollop the remaining turkey mixture over the top; smooth the top. Bake for 30 minutes.

Stir together the tomato paste, balsamic vinegar, and brown sugar. After the loaf has baked for 30 minutes, spread the tomato sauce over the top, then return to the oven for another 30 minutes. Test for doneness with an instant-read thermometer; it's done when it reaches 160°F. Let stand for 5 minutes before slicing.

Keeps for 1 week, tightly covered, in the refrigerator.

EASY BLACK BEAN QUESADILLAS
WITH RASPBERRY-KIWI SALSA

Quesadillas are an incredibly fast and easy meal, and this version swaps healthy, high-fiber beans for most of the cheese, with a delicious result. Whole wheat tortillas become appealingly crispy in the pan, and a fun and fruity salsa completes the feast.

SERVES 6

SALSA

2 large kiwi fruits, peeled and chopped

1 large jalapeño pepper, seeded and chopped

¼ cup fresh cilantro leaves, chopped

1 tablespoon freshly squeezed lime juice

2 large scallions, chopped (white and green parts)

1½ cups fresh raspberries

QUESADILLAS

2 (15-ounce) cans black beans, drained and rinsed, or 3 cups cooked

½ teaspoon ground chipotle powder or chili powder

¾ teaspoon salt

12 (7-inch) whole wheat tortillas

1 cup shredded sharp Cheddar cheese (optional)

For the salsa, combine the kiwi, jalapeño, cilantro, lime, scallions, and raspberries and stir to mix. Reserve.

In a medium bowl, use a fork to mash the beans. Stir in the chipotle powder and salt.

Divide the bean mixture into 6 (⅓-cup) portions and spread each portion onto a tortilla, then top with some cheese, if using, and a second tortilla.

Heat a large cast-iron pan or a nonstick skillet over high heat until hot. Slide each quesadilla into the hot pan and cook until browned, about 1 minute. Use a spatula to flip the quesadilla, then cook on the other side. Slide onto a cutting board and put the next quesadilla into the pan, then cut the hot one into 6 wedges with a chef's knife. Transfer to plates.

Serve warm quesadillas with salsa. Best eaten the day they are made.

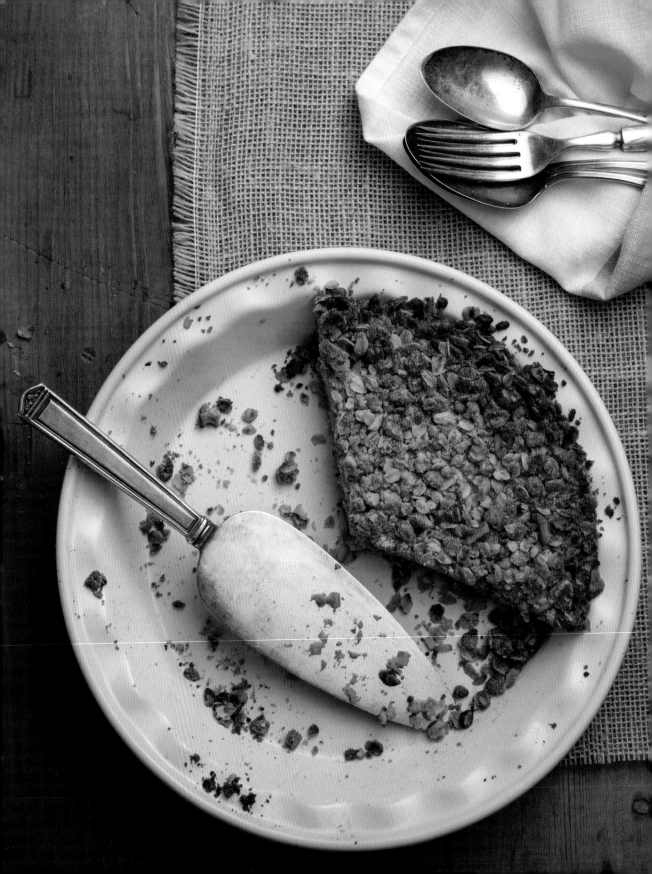

SAVORY STREUSEL SQUASH PIE
with OAT CRUST

Chewy, nutty streusel toppings aren't just for desserts. Savory, herbed, and loaded with sweet squash, this pie will become a family favorite, as a holiday side or a vegetarian main. It also keeps and reheats well, for a squash lover's treat any time of day.

SERVES 8

Canola oil, for the pan

2 pounds kabocha or buttercup squash, baked

2 large onions, chopped

2 tablespoons extra-virgin olive oil

2 tablespoons fresh sage leaves, chopped

2 tablespoons fresh oregano leaves, chopped

6 tablespoons apple juice, divided

1½ teaspoons salt, divided

2 large eggs

2 cups rolled oats

1½ cups whole wheat pastry flour

¼ cup packed light brown sugar

½ cup canola oil

½ cup chopped walnuts

Preheat the oven to 400°F. Lightly oil a 9-inch pie pan. Scoop out the flesh of the baked squash; it should make about 2 cups. Mash the squash in a large bowl. In a large sauté pan over medium heat, sauté the onions in the olive oil until soft and translucent. Keep sautéing and stirring until golden, then add the sage, oregano, 2 tablespoons of the apple juice, and ³/₄ teaspoon of the salt and stir for a minute. Scrape into the bowl with the squash to cool while you prepare the crust. When the squash filling is cool, stir in the eggs.

For the crust and streusel, combine the oats, pastry flour, brown sugar, and remaining ³/₄ teaspoon salt in a large bowl. Stir in the canola oil and remaining apple juice, then measure 1¹/₂ cups of the mixture and press into the oiled pie pan. Press up to just above the rim. Bake for 10 minutes, or until the crust is golden. Into the remaining oat mixture, mix the chopped walnuts.

Spread the squash filling into the cooked crust, level the top, then sprinkle the oat-walnut streusel over the top. Press gently to adhere.

Bake for 40 to 50 minutes, or until the filling is firm when pressed and the streusel is golden brown. Cool for 5 minutes before slicing.

Keeps for 1 week, tightly covered, in the refrigerator.

CHIPOTLE AND AVOCADO GRAIN *AND* TURKEY WRAPS

If you have a piece of leftover turkey or chicken, and some of that lovely grain that you cooked at the beginning of the week, this wrap is the perfect weeknight solution for you. Smoky chipotle and tangy lime-laced salsa mingle with the creamy avocado and chewy grain, giving you an explosion of flavor in every bite.

SERVES 4

SALSA

³/₄ cup chopped grape tomatoes

1 tablespoon freshly squeezed lime juice

1 jalapeño pepper, seeded and chopped

1 medium scallion, chopped (white and green parts)

¹/₂ teaspoon ground cumin

¹/₄ teaspoon salt

2 tablespoons fresh cilantro leaves, chopped

WRAPS

¹/₂ pound turkey breast, cooked and shredded

¹/₂ teaspoon ground chipotle powder

1 cup cooked quinoa or other grain

¹/₄ cup fresh cilantro leaves, chopped

¹/₄ teaspoon salt

1 small avocado

4 large whole wheat tortillas

For the salsa, combine the tomatoes, lime juice, jalapeño, scallion, cumin, salt, and cilantro. Stir gently.

For the wraps, put the turkey in a bowl and sprinkle with the chipotle powder. Reserve. In another bowl, toss the cooked quinoa with the cilantro and salt. Halve the avocado, remove the pit, and mash the avocado coarsely with the quinoa, stirring it in to coat. To assemble the wraps, lay out the tortillas on a cutting board or counter. Arrange a quarter of the turkey in a line down the center of each tortilla, top with quinoa, then spoon a couple tablespoons of salsa on top of the quinoa (leaving the juices behind). Fold in the ends and roll up the wrap. Repeat until all the wraps are done.

Wrap or cover until time to serve. Keeps for 2 days, tightly covered, in the refrigerator.

To serve the wraps, either place seam-side down on a plate and microwave for about 3 minutes until heated through, or spray a large nonstick skillet with oil and pan-toast them over medium heat, seam-side down. Turn and toast the other side until golden. Serve with remaining salsa.

GRAIN-CRUST SPINACH CAULIFLOWER QUICHE

Quiche is a great idea, except that making a pastry crust takes some planning and time. So why not just add cooked whole grains to the mix and let them create a crust, with the bonus of eliminating all the fat and labor that usually go into it? In this tasty pie, cauliflower and spinach combine to give you all the side veggies you might need, too.

SERVES 6

1 tablespoon extra-virgin olive oil, plus more for the pan

2 cups chopped onion

³/₄ cup brown rice

1¹/₂ cups vegetable or chicken stock

¹/₂ teaspoon salt

1 teaspoon dried thyme

¹/₂ teaspoon dried sage, crumbled

2 cups cauliflower florets

1 medium carrot, chopped

2 cups (2 ounces) fresh spinach, chopped

6 ounces Gruyère cheese, shredded (2 cups)

4 large eggs

Preheat the oven to 400°F. Lightly oil a 9-inch pie pan and reserve. Heat a 2-quart heavy saucepan over medium-high heat for a few seconds, then add the oil. Add the onion and sauté, lowering the heat as it softens. Cook until golden and sweet. Add the brown rice and stir, cooking until the grains are hot to the touch and fragrant. Add the stock, salt, thyme, and sage and bring to a boil. Cover tightly and reduce the heat to the lowest setting. Cook for 30 minutes, then quickly add the cauliflower and carrot to the pan, cover again, and let stand for 10 minutes. Uncover and fluff and let cool for about 10 minutes.

In a large bowl, stir the brown rice mixture with the spinach, half of the cheese, and all of the eggs, then scrape into the prepared pie pan. Top with the remaining cheese. Bake for 45 minutes, or until golden on top and firm to the touch. Slice and serve warm.

Keeps for 1 week, tightly covered, in the refrigerator.

SMOKY BACON *and* GRAIN FRITTATA

Make it easy on yourself: just put the meal in a pan and bake it! A couple slices of bacon will flavor a whole frittata, and your farm-fresh eggs can cradle a good-sized serving of wholesome whole grains. Vegetarians can substitute veggie bacon or swap smoked salt for half the regular salt to still reap all the smokiness.

SERVES 4 TO 6

Canola oil, for the pan

2 slices (2 ounces) smoked bacon, chopped

2 garlic cloves, sliced

1 cup broccoli florets

2 ounces kale, stemmed and chopped (3 cups)

8 large eggs

1 teaspoon salt

3/4 cup shredded Parmesan cheese, divided

2 cups cooked wheat berries or other grain

1/2 cup fresh basil leaves, chopped

Preheat the oven to 375°F. Oil a 9-inch pie pan. In a large skillet, cook the bacon until crisp. Use a slotted spatula to transfer the bacon to some paper towels to drain. Pour out the bacon fat as desired, leaving just a little to sauté the vegetables. Put the skillet back on the heat and add the garlic, broccoli, and kale. Stir over medium heat to wilt the kale, about 2 minutes. Take off the heat.

In a large bowl, whisk the eggs with the salt and 1/2 cup of the cheese. Stir in the cooked grain, basil, and bacon and spread into the prepared pie pan. Top with the remaining cheese.

Bake for 35 to 40 minutes, or until the frittata is puffed in the center and the surface is golden. Let cool for 5 minutes before slicing. Keeps for 1 week, tightly covered, in the refrigerator.

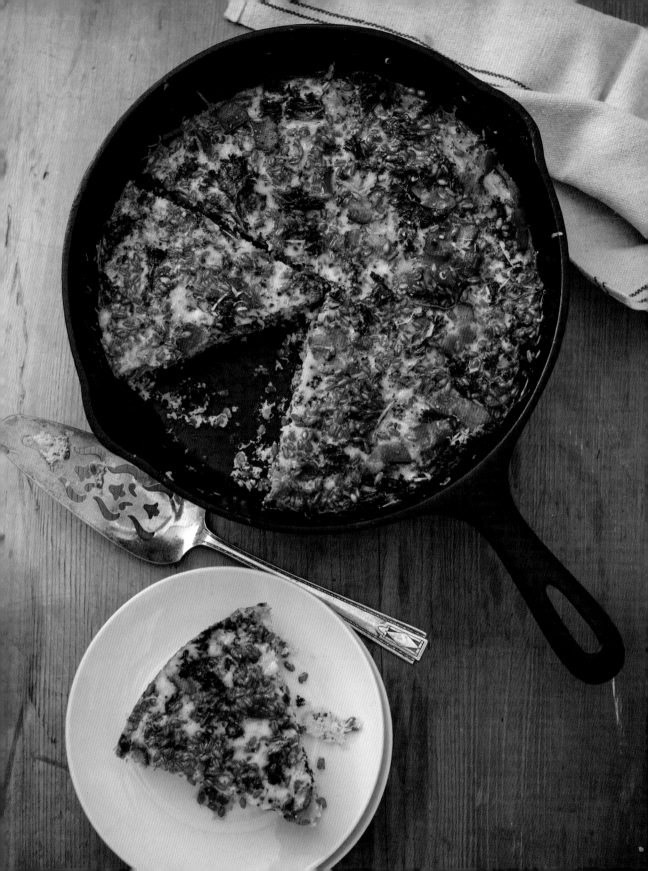

CRUNCHY-CRUMB CHICKEN FINGERS WITH HONEY MUSTARD

It's okay to say that you are just making these for the kids. Just make plenty, because adults love them too. Something about strips of tender white meat coated with crunchy cornmeal and breadcrumbs just calls you to grab one and drag it through the sweet and tangy sauce. Forget the junk food versions—these are made from real chicken and are baked, not fried, so indulge all you want.

SERVES 4 TO 6

Canola oil, for the pan

¾ cup Dijon mustard, divided

½ cup honey

½ cup whole wheat breadcrumbs
(about ½ slice of bread)

½ cup cornmeal

1 tablespoon fresh parsley leaves, chopped

1 tablespoon fresh rosemary leaves, chopped

½ teaspoon salt

¼ teaspoon freshly ground black pepper

1 large egg

3 (8-ounce) skinless, boneless chicken breast halves

Preheat the oven to 400°F. Lightly oil a sheet pan for baking the chicken.

Stir together ½ cup of the Dijon and the honey and reserve.

In a pie pan, combine the breadcrumbs and cornmeal with the parsley, rosemary, salt, and pepper. In another pie pan, whisk the egg and remaining ¼ cup Dijon. Cut each chicken breast into five long, ¾-inch-wide strips. Coat each strip in the egg mixture, then in the crumbs.

Transfer each coated strip to the prepared pan. Bake for 10 minutes, then use a metal spatula to flip the pieces, and bake for 10 minutes more. The strips should be browned in spots.

Serve the hot chicken fingers with the honey mustard for dipping.

Keeps for 3 days, tightly covered, in the refrigerator.

BROWN RICE CALIFORNIA ROLLS WITH SALMON

Sushi would be a perfect food, if only it were made more often with brown rice instead of white. Take matters into your own hands and roll up your favorite fillings with whole grain goodness. Your favorite sushi flavors—like pickled ginger, wasabi, and soy sauce—are all here. For the best results, you will need a sushi-rolling mat and plastic wrap.

SERVES 4

1¼ cups short-grain brown or black rice

2½ cups water

4 teaspoons rice vinegar, plus a dash for rolling

1 teaspoon granulated sugar

½ medium cucumber

1 small carrot

2 medium ripe avocados

4 sheets nori seaweed

4 teaspoons mayonnaise

4 ounces sliced lox

Wasabi, for serving

Pickled ginger, for serving

Soy sauce, for serving

Wash the rice and put it in a heavy 1-quart saucepan with a lid. Add the water, bring to a boil, then reduce the heat to the lowest setting and cover tightly. Cook for 30 to 40 minutes, or until all the water is absorbed. Take off the heat and let stand for 10 minutes, covered. Scrape into a platter or wide bowl to cool slightly. Stir the rice vinegar and sugar together in a small cup, then stir into the rice and cover with a wet towel.

Peel and seed the cucumber, then slice into long, thin strips. Trim the strips to the same length as the width of the nori sheets. Peel the carrot and cut into strips the same way, trimming to the width of the nori. Halve the avocado and remove the pit, then use a paring knife to slice the halves inside the shell. Scoop out with a spoon, making neat slices. Put a bowl of cool water by your cutting board and put a splash of rice vinegar in the water; this is for moistening your fingers. Have a dry towel handy.

If using a rolling mat, wrap it in plastic wrap so that the rice will not stick to the bamboo.

To make your rolls, place a sheet of nori on either a dry cutting board or the rolling mat. Scoop about ³/₄ cup cooled rice onto the sheet of nori. Leaving the top inch uncovered, gently spread the rice across the nori, moistening your fingers as needed to keep the rice from sticking to them. Try to make a very even layer of rice on the nori. On the rice closest to you, smear a teaspoon or so of mayo and place a dab of wasabi. Cover with 1 ounce of lox, about a slice and a half, making an even layer across the bottom. Above that, place a few avocado slices, then two cucumber slices and two carrot strips. Use your fingers to dab a little water across the exposed nori at the top. Using your fingers to hold down the fillings, use your thumbs to roll the nori up, making a neat cylinder. Let the finished roll rest, seam-side down, for a couple of minutes. Repeat with the remaining nori sheets and filling.

Use a sharp knife to slice each roll into 6 pieces, wiping the knife between cuts with a damp cloth. Serve the slices on their sides, with wasabi, pickled ginger, and soy sauce for dipping. Best eaten as soon as it is made.

CORNBREAD-TOPPED CHILI CASSEROLE

Everybody loves a rib-sticking chili, and it can only be better with a topping of fluffy, sunny cornbread. A soon-to-be family favorite, this casserole has the kind of spicy, bold flavors that make whole grains kid-friendly.

SERVES 4 TO 6

1 tablespoon canola oil, plus more for the pan

1 medium onion, chopped

4 ounces (half of an 8-ounce package) cremini
 or button mushrooms, minced

2 garlic cloves, chopped

1 tablespoon chili powder, plus more as needed

¼ cup steel-cut oats

1½ cups vegetable stock or water

1 (15-ounce) can kidney beans, drained and rinsed,
 or 1½ cups cooked

1 (14½-ounce) can diced tomatoes, with juice

½ teaspoon salt

CORNBREAD TOPPING

2 cups cornmeal

2 tablespoons granulated sugar

2 teaspoons baking powder

½ teaspoon baking soda

½ teaspoon salt

1 cup plain yogurt

1 large egg

1 tablespoon canola oil

Lightly oil a 2-quart baking dish. In a large pot, heat the canola oil, then add the onion and sauté, stirring often over medium-high heat. Add the mushrooms and stir, cooking until the mushrooms are dark and shrunken. Add the garlic and chili powder and stir for 1 minute, then add the steel-cut oats and vegetable stock. Bring to a boil, reduce the heat to the lowest setting, and cover tightly. Cook for 15 minutes.

Preheat the oven to 400°F. To the pot, add the kidney beans, tomatoes, and salt. Raise the heat to a boil, then lower to a simmer. Cook for about 5 minutes, or until thickened.

For the topping, while the chili simmers, put the cornmeal, sugar, baking powder, baking soda, and salt in a large bowl. In a cup, whisk together the yogurt, egg, and oil, then stir into the cornmeal mixture.

Transfer the chili to the prepared pan and dollop the cornbread batter over the chili; don't pile it too thickly in the middle. Bake for 30 minutes, or until a toothpick inserted into the cornbread topping in the center of the pan comes out with no wet batter clinging to it.

Serve hot. Once cooled, keeps for 1 week, tightly covered, in the refrigerator.

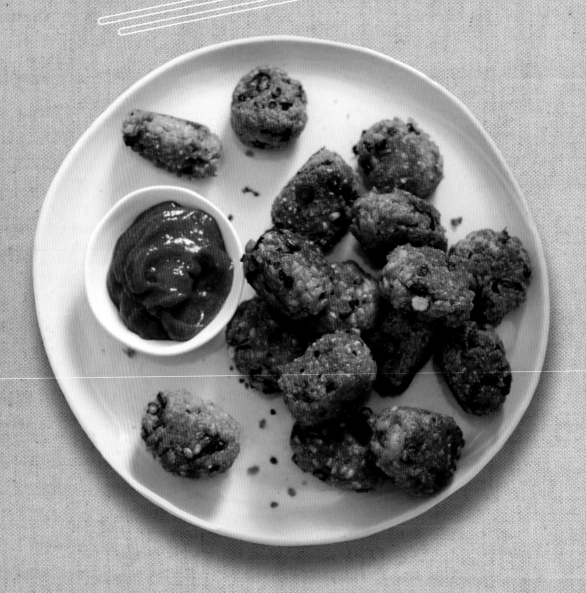

QUICK SNACKS

SUPER POPCORNS

PEANUT BUTTER CORN, CINNAMON CORN *and* PARMESAN CORN

Home-popped corn is one of the healthiest snack foods out there. Whether you pop on the stove or with a popper, these toppings will break you out of a popcorn rut and elevate your corn to treat status.

PEANUT BUTTER CORN

½ cup unpopped popcorn
1 tablespoon canola oil
2 tablespoons unsalted butter
½ cup packed light brown sugar
½ teaspoon vanilla extract
¼ cup apple juice
½ teaspoon salt
¼ cup smooth peanut butter

Preheat the oven to 350°F. Have a large bowl and a parchment-lined sheet pan ready.

In a 4-quart pot, combine the popcorn and oil and place over medium heat. Cover tightly. Shake the pan occasionally as it heats up. When the corn starts popping, shake every minute until the popping slows. Dump the hot popcorn into the large bowl and allow to cool slightly.

In a 1-quart pot, combine the butter and brown sugar and stir over medium heat until the butter is melted. Keep stirring until the mixture boils and is lighter in color, about 2 minutes. Take off the heat and stir in the vanilla, apple juice, and salt (it will bubble up, and the melted sugar will harden in chunks—this is okay), then put back on the heat and return to a boil, stirring constantly. Cook until the sugar is all melted and the mixture is smooth and bubbling, about 2 minutes. Take off the heat and stir in the peanut butter until smooth, then put back on the burner and stir constantly as it comes to a boil again. When the mixture is smooth and slightly thickened, after about 2 minutes, drizzle over the popcorn in the bowl, tossing the popcorn with a heat-safe spatula. Toss the popcorn to coat, then spread on the prepared sheet pan.

Bake the popcorn for about 10 minutes, or just until the peanut butter coating sets and dries. Cool completely on a rack before transferring to an airtight container.

Keeps for 1 week.

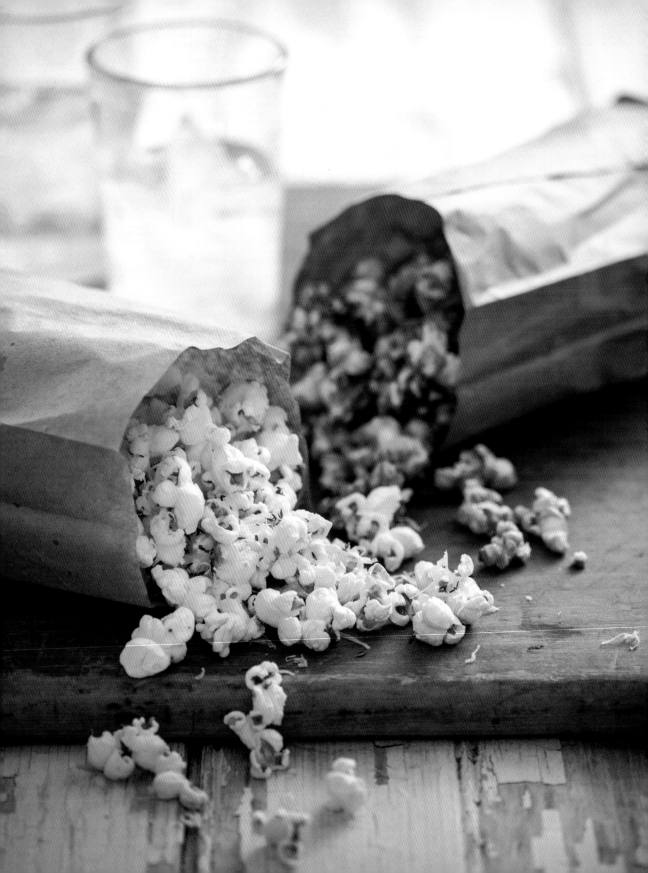

CINNAMON CORN

½ cup unpopped popcorn

1 tablespoon canola oil, plus more
  for the parchment

1 large egg white

½ cup packed light brown sugar

½ teaspoon coarse salt

1 teaspoon cinnamon

Pop the corn (see Peanut Butter Corn recipe for method) and measure out 8 cups popcorn; reserve the rest for another use. Preheat the oven to 300°F. Line a sheet pan with parchment paper and lightly oil the paper. In a medium cup, whisk the egg white, then add the brown sugar, salt, and cinnamon. Drizzle over the popcorn and toss gently to coat. Spread the coated popcorn on the prepared pan. Bake for 15 minutes, stir, and bake for another 15 minutes. Let the popcorn cool on the pan completely before transferring to an airtight container. Keeps for 1 week or more.

PARMESAN CORN

½ cup unpopped popcorn

1 tablespoon canola oil

2 garlic cloves, pressed

2 tablespoons unsalted butter

1 teaspoon dried thyme

½ teaspoon salt

½ cup shredded Parmesan cheese

Pop the corn (see Peanut Butter Corn recipe for method). In a small pan or microwaveable cup, warm the garlic in the butter, then stir in the thyme and salt. While the popcorn is hot, toss with the melted butter mixture and the Parmesan. Serve hot. Transfer cooled leftovers to an airtight container. Keeps for 1 week.

GRAHAM SAMS

GRAHAM CRACKERS WITH CHOCOLATE HAZELNUT, ALMOND-APRICOT SPREAD, MAPLE RICOTTA WITH MINI CHOCOLATE CHIPS, AND APPLES AND CHEDDAR

Ask any parent. Healthy snacks are always in demand, and if you don't plan for them, you might end up snacking on something less than wholesome. Kids and adults alike love graham crackers, despite the fact that they were originally invented as a health food. Whole grains make the crackers wonderfully satisfying and delicious, and adding a tasty topping makes a hearty snack that will keep you going until dinner.

CHOCOLATE HAZELNUT

1 cup hazelnuts, toasted and skinned
1 tablespoon vanilla extract
3 tablespoons unsweetened cocoa powder
3 tablespoons maple syrup
⅛ teaspoon salt
¼ cup plain almond milk or dairy milk

In a food processor, grind and purée the hazelnuts until as smooth as possible. Add the vanilla, cocoa, maple syrup, and salt and process again. Add the almond milk and scrape down, then process to a smooth paste.
Spread on graham crackers.

ALMOND-APRICOT SPREAD

¼ cup almond butter
¼ cup apricot jam

Stir the almond butter and apricot jam together and spread on graham crackers.

MAPLE RICOTTA WITH MINI CHOCOLATE CHIPS

2 tablespoons maple syrup
1 cup ricotta cheese
¼ cup mini chocolate chips

Mix the maple syrup into the ricotta, then stir in the chocolate chips. Spread on graham crackers.

APPLES AND CHEDDAR

1 medium apple, thinly sliced
Pinch of cinnamon
2 ounces sharp Cheddar cheese, thinly sliced

Place the apple slices on graham crackers, sprinkle lightly with cinnamon, then top with the Cheddar.

GRAHAM CRACKER *AND* PUDDING "PIE"

When you really want a dessert but don't want to work too hard, simply blend up this filling and crumble some graham crackers in a pie pan—it's really just that easy. Nobody will notice that the filling is made from healthy tofu, and the hearty crust is all whole grain. If you want to top with melted chocolate drizzle, sliced fruit, berries, or even vanilla yogurt, it will be even more appealing.

SERVES 4

1 (12.3-ounce) aseptic package silken tofu
½ cup maple syrup
4 ounces semisweet chocolate, melted
½ teaspoon vanilla extract
3 sheets whole grain graham crackers
12 large strawberries, sliced

Set out a 3- to 4-cup storage container for the finished pudding. In a food processor, purée the tofu until smooth, stopping to scrape down as necessary. Add the maple syrup, scrape down, and purée again. Add the melted chocolate and very quickly process, before the chocolate has time to harden on the cool tofu. Add the vanilla and process until very well mixed and smooth. Transfer to the storage container. Chill until cold. It will thicken nicely.

To assemble, break about half of the grahams to fit in the bottom of a 9-inch pie pan (use as many graham pieces as it takes to cover it). Dollop half of the chocolate pudding over the grahams and gently spread to fill the pan. Cover with the sliced strawberries, then top with the remaining pudding. Break the remaining grahams into small bits and sprinkle over the pie, patting down as needed to make them flush with the surface. Chill for 1 hour to soften the grahams before serving.

Keeps for 4 days, tightly covered, in the refrigerator.

WHOLE GRAIN CRACKER, CHEX, AND NUT MIXES

CREAMY BUTTERMILK *and* THAI CHILI LIME

The classic party mix starts out with its namesake whole grain cereal, then adds in white bread, white pretzels, and lots of butter. This 100% whole grain version has just a drizzle of butter to stick the snacky coating to the crunchy pieces. Tangy, spicy Thai, and creamy buttermilk flavors make these irresistible.

SERVES 6 TO 8 (MAKES ABOUT 4 CUPS)

CREAMY BUTTERMILK

2 cups Chex or other whole grain cereal

1 cup plain mini rice cakes

1 cup small whole grain pretzels

1 cup small whole wheat crackers

2 tablespoons unsalted butter, melted

3 tablespoons buttermilk powder

¼ teaspoon garlic powder

¼ teaspoon salt

½ cup roasted peanuts, cashews, or almonds

Preheat the oven to 250°F. In a large bowl, combine the cereal, rice cakes, pretzels, and crackers.

Pour the melted butter over the mixture and toss to coat. In a small cup, stir together the buttermilk powder, garlic powder, and salt, then sprinkle over the cereal mixture while tossing to coat.

Spread on a rimmed baking sheet and bake for 45 minutes, stirring every 15.

Let cool, then stir in the nuts. When completely cooled, transfer to airtight bags or tubs. Keeps for 1 week at room temperature.

THAI CHILI LIME

2 cups Chex or other whole grain cereal

1 cup plain mini rice cakes

1 cup small whole grain pretzels

1 cup small whole wheat crackers

2 tablespoons unsalted butter

2 teaspoons freshly grated lime zest

2 teaspoons freshly squeezed lime juice

1 tablespoon tamari or soy sauce

1 garlic clove, pressed

1 teaspoon Sriracha sauce

½ cup roasted peanuts or cashews

Preheat the oven to 250°F. In a large bowl, combine the cereal, rice cakes, pretzels, and crackers.

Melt the butter in a microwave safe cup. Add lime zest and juice, tamari, garlic, and Sriracha and heat for 1 minute. Stir and heat again just until bubbling slightly. Pour over the cereal mixture in the bowl and use a spatula to toss to coat.

Spread on a baking sheet and bake for 45 minutes, stirring every 15.

Let cool, then stir in the nuts. When completely cooled, transfer to airtight bags or tubs. Keeps for 1 week at room temperature.

CINNAMON TOASTS *WITH* YOGURT DIP

Bagel chips and Melba toast are both packaged foods that are really just ways to use up old bread. Why not make these easy, crispy toast dippers and dip them in some yogurt? This is a great way to use up any extra bread from your No-Knead "Stealth" loaf (page 67). Easy to pack in a lunchbox or backpack, along with a jar of fruity dip—you can't miss.

SERVES 6

2 large egg whites

6 pieces whole wheat bread

2 tablespoons granulated sugar

1½ teaspoons cinnamon

DIP

½ cup chopped fruit, such as kiwi, banana, berries, or apples

1 cup vanilla yogurt

Preheat the oven to 300°F. Lightly coat a sheet pan with vegetable oil spray. In a wide, flat bowl, whisk the egg whites. Stack the bread and slice into three long slices per slice of bread. Dip each in the egg white mixture, scraping off the excess on the side of the bowl. Place on the sprayed pan.

Combine the sugar and cinnamon. Sprinkle half of the cinnamon sugar on the bread pieces, then carefully turn them over, and sprinkle the remaining cinnamon sugar on the other side.

Bake for 15 minutes, then use a metal spatula to flip the bread pieces. Bake for 15 minutes longer, or until crisp and dry.

Cool on the pan on a rack for 5 minutes, then transfer the pieces to the rack. Let cool completely before storing in an airtight container. Keeps for 1 week, tightly covered, at room temperature.

For the dip: Stir the fruit into the yogurt and serve with cinnamon toasts.

BAKED CORN CHIPS
WITH EASY EDAMAME HUMMUS

Freshly baked, lightly spiced corn chips will give bagged chips a run for the money, with no deep-fat frying in mystery oils. Add a creamy, pale green version of the familiar hummus, and you have a hearty, fiber-filled snack that will hold you over until dinnertime.

SERVES 4 (MAKES ABOUT 4 CUPS)

1 tablespoon canola oil

6 corn tortillas

Salt

HUMMUS

SERVES 4 (MAKES 1½ CUPS)

1 garlic clove

1 cup frozen edamame, thawed

½ cup tahini

¼ cup freshly squeezed lemon juice

⅓ cup water

½ teaspoon salt, or more to taste

2 tablespoons extra-virgin olive oil (optional)

Preheat the oven to 350°F. Measure the canola oil into a cup. Use a pastry brush to lightly brush each tortilla on both sides with the oil, then stack them on a cutting board. Use a sharp chef's knife to cut the tortillas into 6 wedges. Brush any remaining oil on two sheet pans and distribute the corn tortillas over the pans. Sprinkle with salt.

Bake for 15 minutes, switching the pans in the oven halfway through. The chips will be golden brown in spots, puffed, and crisp. Cool on the pans on racks.

For the hummus, drop the garlic into a food processor with the machine running. Scrape down, then add the edamame and process to chop as finely as possible. Add the tahini, lemon juice, water, and salt and process. Add the olive oil, if desired, and blend to mix.

The chips keep for 1 week, tightly sealed, and the hummus keeps for 4 days, tightly covered, in the refrigerator.

YOGURT-GRANOLA PARFAIT
wiᵗʰ SEASONAL FRUIT

Now that you have your fabulous homemade granola, make an easy layered snack with yogurt and fruit. Creamy, crunchy, sweet, and tangy, this parfait makes a little look like a lot.

SERVES 1

¾ cup vanilla yogurt

½ cup pan-toasted or other granola
  (see recipes on pages 31–33)

1 medium nectarine, pear, apple, or banana, sliced

¼ cup berries

Chia seeds, flax seeds, or hemp seeds (optional)

Build your parfait in a glass or bowl that holds 1³/₄ cups. Measure ¹/₂ cup of the yogurt into the glass. Sprinkle in ¹/₄ cup granola, then add the sliced fruit. Add the remaining yogurt, the berries, and the remaining granola.

If desired, add 1 tablespoon of the optional seeds to the first layer of granola.

Cover your parfait with plastic wrap, and it will keep for 4 days in the refrigerator.

WHOLE WHEAT PITA PIZZAS

Whole wheat pitas are the simplest way to make a snack pizza—just top and bake. You can even microwave them if you want. Keep pitas in your fridge or freezer for instant access when the hungries hit!

SERVES 4

12 ounces fresh spinach or other green, such as kale
  or chard, tough stems removed
1 teaspoon extra-virgin olive oil
Pinch of salt
4 whole wheat pitas
1 cup (8 ounces) ricotta cheese
20 medium grape tomatoes, halved
¼ cup shredded Parmesan cheese

Preheat the oven to 425°F. Bring a pot of water to a boil. Drop the spinach in and stir. Cook for about 2 minutes, or until softened, then drain, rinse with cold water, and wring out until very dry. Chop the drained greens, then put in a medium bowl and toss with the olive oil and salt.

Assemble the pizzas. Place the pitas on two sheet pans and among the ricotta between the pitas, spreading to cover. Divide the greens among the four pitas, patting down. Cover with halved tomatoes and sprinkle with Parmesan cheese.

Bake for 15 minutes, or until the pitas are crisp and there are golden spots on the cheese. Serve immediately.

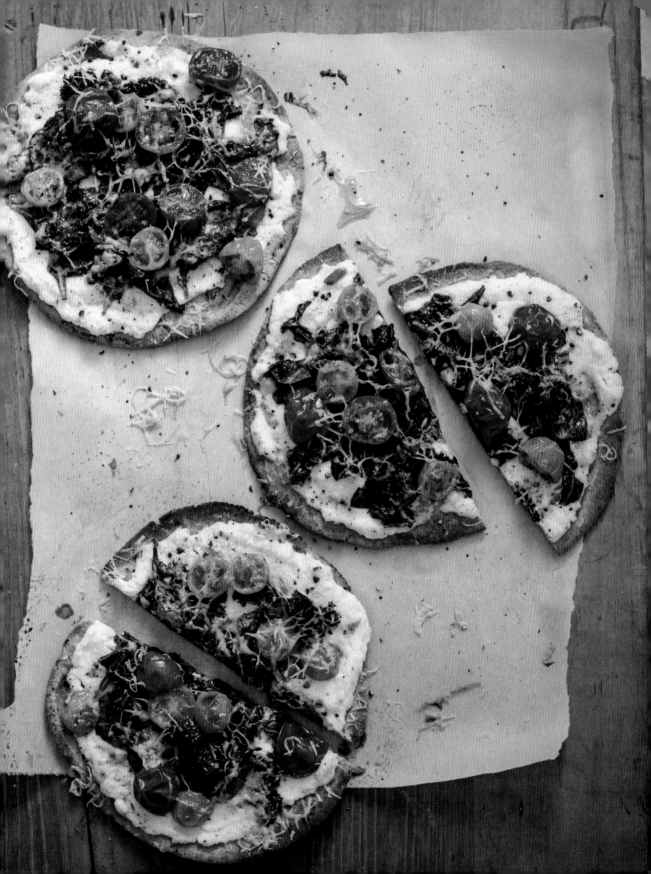

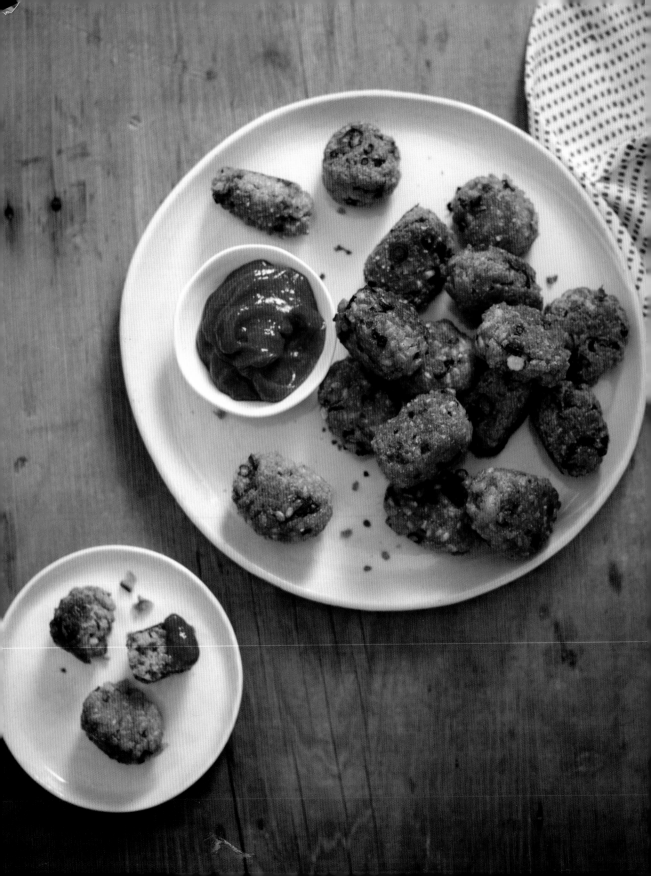

LEFTOVER-GRAIN SCALLION CAKES
with CURRY KETCHUP

Once you have those cooked grains in the fridge, you are set to make these little pancakes, puffed and golden and chock-full of your favorite grain. A simple dip of ketchup with curry will make them irresistible.

SERVES 4 TO 6 (MAKES ABOUT 20)

1/2 cup ketchup

2 teaspoons curry powder

1/4 cup cornmeal

1/2 cup white whole wheat flour

1 teaspoon ground cumin

1 teaspoon ground coriander

1/2 teaspoon freshly ground black pepper

1/2 teaspoon baking powder

1/2 teaspoon baking soda

1/2 teaspoon salt

3/4 cup nonfat plain yogurt

1 tablespoon canola oil, plus more for frying

1 large egg

2 cups cooked grain

4 medium scallions, chopped (white and green parts)

Preheat the oven to 250°F to hold the finished fritters for serving, if desired. Line an oven-safe plate with paper towels for draining. Stir together the ketchup and curry powder in a small bowl.

In a large bowl, whisk together the cornmeal, flour, cumin, coriander, pepper, baking powder, baking soda, and salt. In a medium bowl, whisk the yogurt, canola oil, and egg until mixed. Place a large skillet (or two) over medium-high heat and drizzle in canola oil to cover the bottom(s). Quickly stir the yogurt mixture into the cornmeal mixture, just until combined, then stir in the cooked grain and scallions.

When the pan is hot and the oil is shimmery, scoop 2-tablespoon-sized portions of batter into the pan, patting the tops lightly to level. Leave 1/2 inch between cakes. When the oil starts to sizzle again, lower the heat to medium. When they start to bubble in the centers and look firm and golden around the edges, flip with a metal spatula. Cook on the other side for a couple of minutes, then transfer to the prepared plate. Continue until all the cakes are done.

Serve the cakes hot, with curry ketchup for dipping.

The cakes keep for 4 days, tightly covered, in the refrigerator.

RICE CAKE TUNA MELTS

For the ultimate pantry snack, try topping your crunchy rice cake with some canned tuna (or salmon, if you prefer) and a little cheese. Quick, crunchy, filling, and full of essential fatty acids.

SERVES 2

1 (7.5-ounce) can water-packed
   tuna or salmon, drained

2 tablespoons minced celery

1 medium scallion, chopped
   (white and green parts)

1 tablespoon fresh parsley leaves, chopped

3 tablespoons plain Greek yogurt

1 tablespoon Dijon mustard

4 large grape tomatoes, sliced

1½ ounces Havarti cheese,
   cut into 6 thin slices

2 plain rice cakes

Set an oven rack 6 inches from the broiler and preheat the broiler.

In a medium bowl, combine the tuna, celery, scallion, parsley, yogurt, and Dijon and stir to mix. Spread the tuna mixture on the rice cakes, then top with tomato slices and cheese.

Broil, monitoring constantly, for 1 to 2 minutes, or until the cheese is melted, bubbly, and browned.

Serve immediately.

SAVORY OATMEAL COOKIES WITH CHEDDAR

A savory cookie? Absolutely! With just a hint of sweetness and some zingy crystallized ginger and cranberries, these cookies are just as good with a glass of wine as with a glass of cold milk. Chunks of Cheddar make them a sustaining snack, great for toting along on your busy day.

SERVES 24 (MAKES 24 COOKIES)

1 cup whole wheat pastry flour

1 teaspoon dried sage

½ teaspoon dried thyme

½ teaspoon baking soda

½ teaspoon salt

1½ cups rolled oats

½ cup (1 stick) unsalted butter

2 large eggs

¼ cup packed light brown sugar

1 teaspoon vanilla extract

½ cup crystallized ginger, chopped

½ cup dried cranberries

4 ounces sharp Cheddar cheese, diced

Preheat the oven to 375°F. Line two baking sheets with parchment paper. In a large bowl, whisk together the flour, sage, thyme, baking soda, salt, and oats.

In the bowl of a stand mixer or a large bowl, beat the butter until fluffy, then beat in the eggs and brown sugar. Beat in the vanilla. Beat the flour mixture into the butter mixture and then fold in the ginger, cranberries, and Cheddar on low speed. Scoop ¼-cup portions and place them 2 inches apart on the prepared pans. Wet your palms and flatten the cookies slightly.

Bake for 10 minutes, then switch the pans and bake for 8 minutes more. The cookies will be golden brown. Transfer to a rack to cool.

Keeps for 1 week, tightly covered, in the refrigerator.

DESSERTS

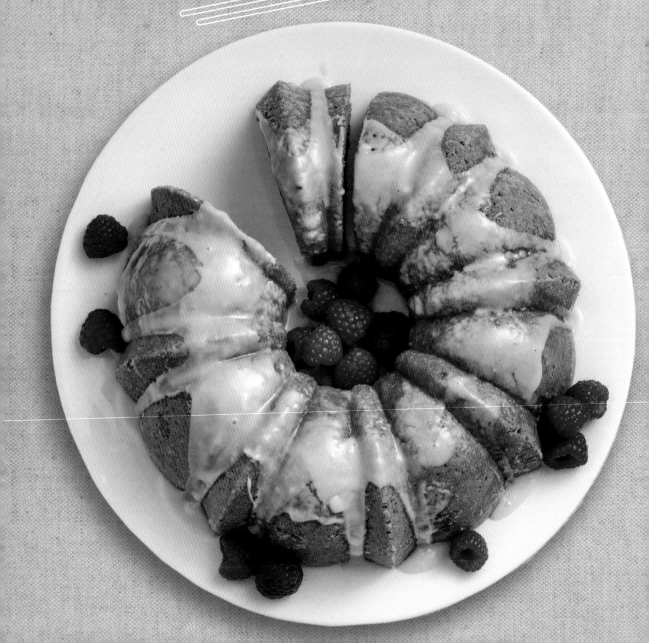

GRANOLA BARK

Have you heard? Dark chocolate is a health food! This incredibly easy and fast little treat is a great way to eat chocolate. Get your daily dose of antioxidants and happiness-inducing chemicals, with a topping of crunchy whole grain granola. Of course, if you prefer milk chocolate, you can use that, too.

SERVES 8

½ cup granola (see recipes on pages 31–33)
8 ounces semisweet chocolate

Line a 9-inch square baking pan with waxed paper, cutting the paper so that the ends go up and slightly over two sides of the pan and can be used as handles to lift the finished bark from the pan. Measure the granola and reserve. In a microwave-safe bowl in the microwave, or over a double boiler, melt the chocolate. Spread the chocolate in the prepared pan. Sprinkle the granola evenly over the chocolate and tap down lightly to nestle the chunks into the chocolate. Chill until firm.

When the chocolate is firm, break the bark into your desired-sized pieces. Keeps for 2 weeks, in a tightly covered storage tub or resealable bag, in a cool place or the refrigerator.

GRANOLA BRITTLE CHUNKS

Peanut brittle is a classic treat around the holidays, but why not branch out with this whole grain version? It's still dessert, and you'll still get to enjoy the buttery crunch of the brittle you remember from childhood, but because this treat is full of fiber and oaty goodness, you will be satiated after just a few bites.

SERVES 12

GRANOLA

4 cups rolled oats

¼ teaspoon salt

¼ cup canola oil, plus more for the pan

¼ cup honey

BRITTLE

2 cups granulated sugar

½ cup water

½ cup (1 stick) unsalted butter, plus more for the spoon

¼ cup honey

½ teaspoon baking soda

First, make the granola. Preheat the oven to 300°F and lightly oil a sheet pan. In a large bowl, combine the oats and salt. In a cup, stir together the oil and honey, then stir into the oats. Spread on the sheet pan and bake for 20 minutes. Stir, then bake for 20 minutes more. Stir, then bake for a final 20 minutes. Cool on a rack.

For the brittle: Line a large rimmed sheet pan with parchment paper and reserve. Butter the back of a large wooden or metal spoon for spreading the hot brittle in the pan.

In a 2-quart saucepan, combine the sugar, water, butter, and honey and bring to a boil. Cook over medium-high heat, stirring occasionally, until the caramel is light brown and registers 300°F on a candy thermometer, about 10 minutes. Remove from the heat and carefully stir in the baking soda. The mixture will bubble. Stir in the granola, then immediately scrape the brittle onto the prepared sheet pan. Using the back of the buttered spoon, spread the brittle into a thin, even layer. You have to move quickly to get it to about ½ inch thick. Let cool completely, about 30 minutes.

Break the brittle into large shards. Keeps for 2 weeks in airtight containers at room temperature.

"RAW" COOKIE DOUGH BITES

Admit it. You have eaten raw cookie dough. It's become a popular ice cream add-in and even a cocktail flavor, so cookie dough's yum factor cannot be denied. With this recipe, you can have all the gooey, forbidden flavor of chocolate chip cookie dough, with none of the raw eggs. The whole grain flour is the last thing your snackers will notice.

SERVES 10 (MAKES 20 BITES)

2 tablespoons unsalted butter, at room temperature
½ cup packed light brown sugar
½ teaspoon vanilla extract
¼ cup plain Greek yogurt (nonfat is fine)
½ cup white whole wheat flour
½ cup chocolate chips
¼ cup buckwheat groats
10 ounces chocolate, for coating (optional)

In the bowl of a stand mixer or a large bowl, cream the butter. Add the brown sugar and beat until well mixed. Add the vanilla and yogurt and beat, scraping down as necessary, until well mixed. Mix in the flour, and when combined, stir in the chocolate chips and groats.

Scrape the dough into a storage container and chill for 30 minutes or overnight. Scoop tablespoon-sized portions and form into balls. Place on a plate and chill, tightly covered, until time to serve.

For the optional chocolate coating, melt the chocolate in a double boiler, then let cool to room temperature. Line a sheet pan with parchment or waxed paper. Use a fork to lower each chilled cookie dough ball into the chocolate, then tap the fork on the side of the pan to remove excess chocolate. Place on the lined pan and chill until set.

Keeps for 1 week, tightly covered, in the refrigerator.

QUICK STOVETOP NECTARINE-BERRY CRUMBLE

Doesn't it always seem that fruit is best for baking on the hottest days of summer? Don't skip that crisp because you don't want to crank up the oven. In this stovetop wonder, you will make the fruity filling in one pan, toast up a crunchy topping in another, and then meld the two. All of the appeal of your favorite baked dessert, minus the hot oven. Adorn it with a scoop of ice cream, and you will have a truly classic dessert.

SERVES 8

4 large nectarines
5 tablespoons unsalted butter, divided
2 cups fresh blueberries or raspberries
1 cup packed light brown sugar, divided
2 tablespoons water
1 tablespoon arrowroot
2 cups rolled oats
2 teaspoons cinnamon
¼ teaspoon salt

You will need a 10- to 12-inch cast-iron skillet and another large sauté pan. Slice the nectarines, then melt 1 tablespoon of the butter in the cast-iron skillet over medium heat. Add the nectarines and stir. Cook, stirring, until the fruit is soft and juicy, about 3 minutes. Stir in the blueberries and cook for 1 minute. Add ¼ cup of the brown sugar and stir until syrupy. Whisk the water and arrowroot together in a cup and stir into the simmering fruit. Take the pan off the heat. If desired, transfer the fruit to a 9-inch pie pan, or leave it in the cast-iron pan.

While you are cooking the fruit, put the oats in the large sauté pan and swirl over medium-high heat. When the oats start to feel hot to the touch and smell a little toasty, lower the heat so they don't burn. When the oats are lightly golden, add the remaining ¾ cup brown sugar, cinnamon, and salt and swirl and stir constantly until the sugar is melted. Add the remaining 4 tablespoons butter and take off the heat, stirring to coat the oats with butter. Put back over the heat and stir for a few more seconds.

Distribute the oat mixture over the hot fruit mixture, and if you are leaving the fruit in the cast-iron pan, put the pan back on the heat and bring it to a bubble undisturbed. Take the pan off the heat again and let cool for 10 minutes before serving.

If you are using a pie pan, tap the pan on the counter to settle the topping. Cool slightly before serving. Keeps for 4 days, tightly covered, in the refrigerator.

OATMEAL *AND* MIXED-FRUIT JUMBO COOKIES

Oatmeal cookies are one of the most popular kinds of home-baked cookie, winning the hearts of generations of hungry kids. These are super oaty and packed with chewy dried fruit for a satisfying and sweet cookie that will never get traded at lunch. For truly jumbo cookies, use the $1/2$-cup measure to portion out the dough, or use the $1/4$-cup measure to make regular-sized cookies.

SERVES 6 TO 8 (MAKES 6 OR 12 COOKIES)

$1\frac{1}{2}$ cups rolled oats
1 cup whole wheat pastry flour
1 teaspoon baking soda
$\frac{1}{2}$ teaspoon salt
1 teaspoon cinnamon
$\frac{1}{4}$ cup canola oil
$\frac{1}{2}$ cup honey
1 tablespoon freshly grated orange zest
2 tablespoons freshly squeezed orange juice
1 teaspoon vanilla extract
$\frac{1}{2}$ cup raisins
$\frac{1}{2}$ cup dried apricots, chopped
$\frac{1}{2}$ cup dried cherries

Preheat the oven to 375°F. Line a large baking sheet with parchment paper. In a large bowl, combine the oats, flour, baking soda, salt, and cinnamon. In a medium bowl, combine the canola oil, honey, orange zest and juice, and vanilla. Stir the honey mixture into the oat mixture until well combined, then stir in the fruit.

Use either a $1/2$-cup or $1/4$-cup measure to scoop the dough onto the parchment-lined pan, leaving 2 inches between the portions of dough. Wet your palms with water and gently flatten the dough rounds to about $3/4$ inch thick, just to make them even. Bake for 16 minutes for the jumbo cookies or 12 minutes for the smaller cookies, turning the pan in the oven at the 8- or 6-minute mark.

Cool completely on the pan on a rack and then transfer the cookies to the rack. Keeps for 1 week in an airtight container at room temperature.

CHEWY CHOCOLATE COOKIES

These cookies are light and chewy, with no butter but plenty of chocolate flavor. The whole grain flour and oats are just added interest in a cookie that you will enjoy with a glass of milk or a cup of coffee, any time of day.

SERVES 18 (MAKES 18 COOKIES)

6 tablespoons white whole wheat flour

½ cup whole wheat pastry flour

2 tablespoons unsweetened cocoa powder

¼ teaspoon baking soda

¼ teaspoon salt

1 large egg

¾ cup packed light brown sugar

1 teaspoon vanilla extract

1 ounce unsweetened chocolate

½ cup rolled oats

Position racks in the upper and lower thirds of the oven and preheat to 375°F. Line two large baking sheets with parchment paper.

In a large bowl, combine the white whole wheat flour, whole wheat pastry flour, cocoa, baking soda, and salt. Whisk to mix. In a medium bowl, whisk the egg and brown sugar until light, about 1 minute. Whisk in the vanilla. Melt the chocolate in the microwave or in a double boiler. Scrape the chocolate into the egg mixture and quickly whisk in. Stir the egg mixture into the flour mixture, and when combined, stir in the oats.

Scoop heaping tablespoon-sized portions onto the lined pans, leaving 2 inches between the portions of dough.

Bake for 6 minutes, then switch the positions of the pans and bake for 6 minutes more. The cookies will be puffed and crackled on top. Cool on the baking sheets on a rack for 5 minutes before using a metal spatula to transfer the cookies to the rack. Cool completely.

Keeps for 1 week in an airtight container at room temperature.

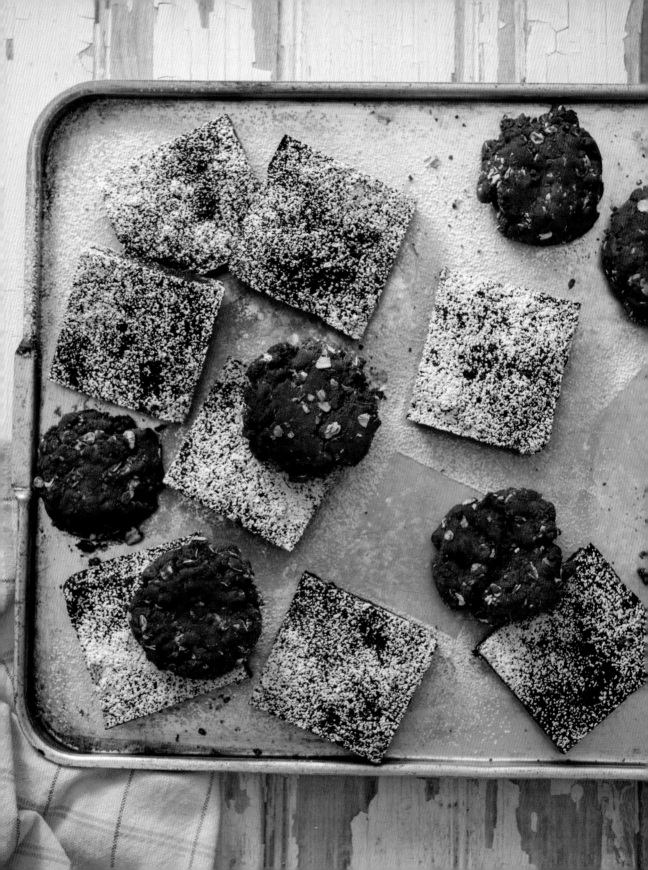

LIGHT BUCKWHEAT BROWNIES

Brownies don't have to be dripping with butter to be good. Take advantage of applesauce and other healthy ingredients for a satisfyingly chocolaty brownie, with barely a trace of fat. These are embellished with a little earthy buckwheat flour for a truly interesting treat.

SERVES 12

Canola oil, for the pan

1 cup applesauce, drained to about ⅔ cup (see directions below)

1 cup packed light brown sugar

1 teaspoon vanilla extract

2 large eggs

½ cup nonfat plain Greek yogurt

½ cup buckwheat flour

¾ cup whole wheat pastry flour

¾ cup unsweetened cocoa powder

½ teaspoon baking soda

½ teaspoon salt

½ cup miniature chocolate chips (optional)

Confectioners' sugar, for dusting

Preheat the oven to 350°F. Oil a 9-inch square baking pan and reserve.

If you have a yogurt strainer, drain the applesauce for 15 minutes. If not, spread the applesauce on a five-fold thickness of paper towels, let the towels absorb water from the sauce, and then scrape the remaining apple purée carefully into a large bowl. Stir in the sugar, vanilla, and eggs until smoothly mixed, then beat in the yogurt.

In another bowl, whisk together the flours, cocoa, baking soda, and salt. Stir into the wet mixture just until moistened. Stir in the chocolate chips, if using.

Scrape into the prepared pan and smooth the top. Bake for 20 to 25 minutes, or until done around the edges but still quite moist in the middle. Cool completely (or chill for neater slices) before slicing into 2-inch brownies. Dust with confectioners' sugar and serve.

Keeps for 1 week, tightly covered, at room temperature or in the refrigerator.

APPLE BUTTER-SWIRL CUPCAKES
WITH CIDER GLAZE

Apple butter is the magic ingredient here, with a swirl that is thick and rich and redolent of spice. Twirl it into these tender cupcakes and drizzle them with an easy apple cider glaze, and you'll never miss the frosting.

SERVES 12 (MAKES 12 CUPCAKES)

1½ cups whole wheat pastry flour

1 cup unbleached flour

1 teaspoon baking powder

1 teaspoon baking soda

½ teaspoon salt

¾ cup maple syrup

¾ cup almond milk or other milk

2 teaspoons rice vinegar

⅓ cup canola oil, plus more for the pan

½ cup apple butter, plus more as needed

GLAZE

½ cup confectioners' sugar

1½ tablespoons apple cider

Preheat the oven to 350°F. Line 12 muffin cups with paper liners and oil the top of the pan so the cupcake tops won't stick.

In a large bowl, combine the flours, baking powder, baking soda, and salt and stir well.

In a medium bowl, stir together the maple syrup, milk, vinegar, and canola oil.

Stir the wet mixture into the dry ingredients, mixing until there are no lumps. Scoop about 3 tablespoons batter into each muffin cup, then drop a teaspoon of apple butter in and swirl. Top with more batter, add another teaspoon of apple butter, and swirl.

Bake for about 20 minutes, or until a toothpick inserted in the center of a cupcake comes out with no wet batter clinging to it. Cool on a rack for 5 minutes before carefully transferring the cupcakes to the rack to cool completely.

For the glaze, put the confectioners' sugar in a bowl or cup and stir in the cider with a fork. Use the fork to drizzle glaze on the cupcakes. Let the glaze dry before storing or serving.

Keeps for 1 week in an airtight container at room temperature, but best in the refrigerator.

PEANUT BUTTER CAKE
WITH CHOCOLATE FROSTING

Two great tastes that taste great together, peanut butter and chocolate will always be in style. In this fluffy cake, the familiar taste of peanut butter helps cover for the whole wheat, and a completely decadent yogurt-based chocolate frosting takes it over the top. I love this made with very dark chocolate and plain yogurt, but if you are making it for kids, you might try using 60% cacao chocolate and vanilla yogurt.

SERVES 12

1½ cups whole wheat pastry flour
¾ cup packed light brown sugar
1 teaspoon baking powder
½ teaspoon baking soda
½ teaspoon salt
½ cup smooth peanut butter
¼ cup canola oil, plus more for the pan
2 large eggs

¾ cup milk
1 teaspoon vanilla extract

FROSTING

6 ounces dark chocolate
1½ cups plain Greek yogurt, at room temperature
1 teaspoon vanilla extract

Preheat the oven to 350°F. Lightly oil a 9-inch square baking pan.

In a large bowl, combine the flour and brown sugar, breaking up any lumps of sugar with your fingers. Add the baking powder, baking soda, and salt and whisk to blend.

In a medium bowl, stir together the peanut butter, canola oil, eggs, milk, and vanilla until smooth. Quickly stir the peanut butter mixture into the flour mixture, then scrape the batter into the prepared pan.

Bake for 25 to 30 minutes, or until a toothpick inserted in the center of the pan comes out with only a few moist crumbs attached.

Cool the cake in the pan on a rack.

To make the frosting, melt the chocolate in a double boiler or in the microwave. While the chocolate is hot and liquid, dump in the yogurt and vanilla and stir quickly to mix. When smooth, spread on the cake and chill.

Keeps for 4 days, tightly covered, in the refrigerator.

CHERRY-ALMOND GRAIN PUDDING

Rice pudding has always been a comfort food but still classy enough to be offered in gourmet versions in the best of restaurants. The formula is simple: just bake your rice in a tasty custard studded with fruit. You can make this with just about any grain, although short-grain red rice will provide a wonderful, pillowy chewiness to the dish.

SERVES 6

Canola oil, for the pan
3 large eggs
1 cup almond milk or other milk
½ cup honey
1 teaspoon vanilla extract
1 teaspoon almond extract
¼ teaspoon salt
3 cups cooked red rice or other grain (1 cup uncooked)
1 cup dried cherries
¼ cup slivered almonds
Whipped cream, for serving (optional)

Preheat the oven to 350°F. Lightly oil a 2-quart casserole pan.

In a medium bowl, whisk the eggs, then whisk in the almond milk, honey, vanilla, almond extract, and salt. Stir in the cooked grain and cherries, then transfer to the prepared baking dish. Sprinkle the almond slivers evenly over the top.

Bake for 50 to 60 minutes, or until a toothpick inserted in the center comes out with no wet batter on it. Serve warm or chilled and topped with whipped cream, if desired.

Once cooled, keeps for 1 week, tightly covered, in the refrigerator.

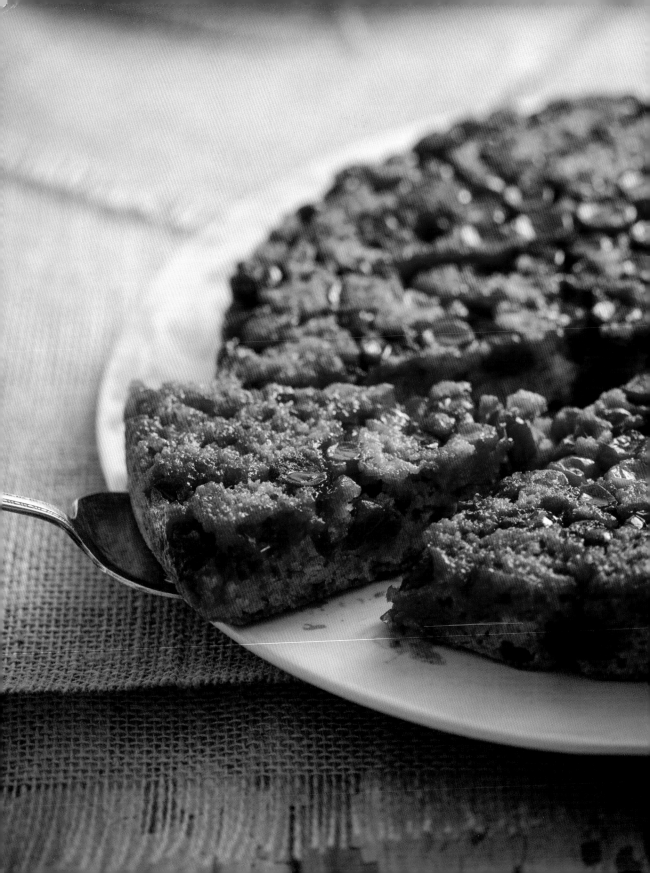

CRANBERRY CORNMEAL UPSIDE-DOWN CAKE

Cranberries make a bright topping for this luscious cake, which is perfect for a fall dessert or a change from the usual pumpkin pie at Thanksgiving. Sweet, toothsome cornmeal makes the cake sturdy enough to stand up to the tangy, buttery berry topping, with delicious results.

SERVES 10

6 tablespoons unsalted butter

1 cup packed light brown sugar

2 cups cranberries, fresh or frozen

1 cup medium-grind cornmeal

3/4 cup whole wheat pastry flour

1/2 cup granulated sugar

2 tablespoons freshly grated orange zest

1/2 teaspoon baking powder

1/2 teaspoon baking soda

1/4 teaspoon salt

1/4 cup canola oil

1 large egg

3/4 cup plain yogurt

1 teaspoon vanilla extract

Preheat the oven to 375°F. Wrap an 11-inch round springform pan with foil so that if any butter leaks out, it won't burn in the oven. Put the butter in the pan and place the pan in the oven for 5 to 10 minutes as the oven heats up. Remove from the oven and tilt the pan to cover evenly with melted butter. Sprinkle the brown sugar evenly in the pan and distribute the cranberries evenly over that. Reserve.

In a large bowl, combine the cornmeal, flour, granulated sugar, zest, baking powder, baking soda, and salt. In a medium bowl, whisk together the canola oil, egg, yogurt, and vanilla.

Mix the wet ingredients into the dry ingredients, stirring until well combined. Scrape the batter evenly over the cranberries in the pan.

Bake for about 45 minutes, or until a toothpick inserted in the center of the cake comes out with moist crumbs but no raw batter on it.

Cool for 5 minutes in the pan on a rack. Place a plate over the cake, and holding them together firmly, flip to invert the cake onto the plate. If any topping stays in the pan, quickly pick it out with a butter knife and fill it in any gaps on the cake. Let cool completely before serving.

Keeps for 1 week, tightly covered, in the refrigerator.

ORANGE-RASPBERRY BUNDT

Bundt cakes are great for beginning bakers, since the tube shape bakes the batter evenly, and you don't have to fuss with frosting layers. This is a real cake with a moist, buttery crumb and a tangy tender texture. The orange zest lifts it to another level, and the juicy berries punctuate every few bites.

SERVES 12

2¼ cups plus 2 teaspoons whole wheat pastry flour, divided, plus more for the pan

1 teaspoon baking powder

1 teaspoon baking soda

½ teaspoon salt

2 tablespoons freshly grated orange zest (from about 1 large navel orange)

½ cup (1 stick) unsalted butter, at room temperature, plus more for the pan

1 cup packed light brown sugar

2 large eggs

1½ cups nonfat plain Greek yogurt

1 teaspoon vanilla extract

4 tablespoons freshly squeezed orange juice, divided (from about 1 large navel orange)

1 cup fresh raspberries

1 cup confectioners' sugar

Preheat the oven to 350°F. Grease and flour a Bundt pan.

In a medium bowl, whisk 2¼ cups of the flour with the baking powder, baking soda, salt, and orange zest.

In the bowl of a stand mixer or in a large bowl, beat the butter until fluffy. Beat in the brown sugar, then beat in the eggs. In a medium bowl, combine the yogurt, vanilla, and 2 tablespoons of the orange juice. Add one third of the flour mixture to the butter mixture, beating on low, then add half of the yogurt mixture, another third of the flour mixture, the remaining yogurt mixture, and the last of the flour mixture. Scrape the bowl well, making sure all the butter is incorporated.

Toss the raspberries with the remaining 2 teaspoons flour to coat.

Scrape two thirds of the batter into the prepared pan and drop the raspberries evenly in the center of the batter, then dollop over the remaining batter. Smooth the top with a spatula. Bake for 50 to 55 minutes, or until deep golden brown and a toothpick inserted in the center of the cake comes out with no wet batter clinging to it. Cool the cake in the pan on a rack until completely cool, then run a paring knife between the cake and the pan, place a serving plate on top, and invert the cake.

Whisk together the confectioners' sugar and remaining 2 tablespoons orange juice to make a pourable glaze. If you don't have quite enough juice, stir in a little milk or water just until it will drizzle. Pour over the cooled cake and let set for 30 minutes before cutting.

Keeps for 1 week, tightly covered, in the refrigerator.

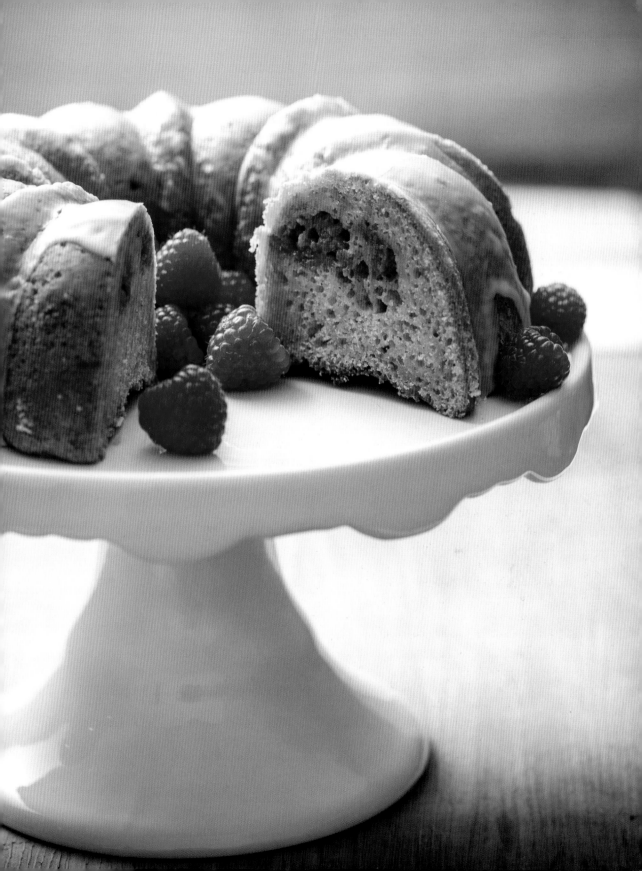

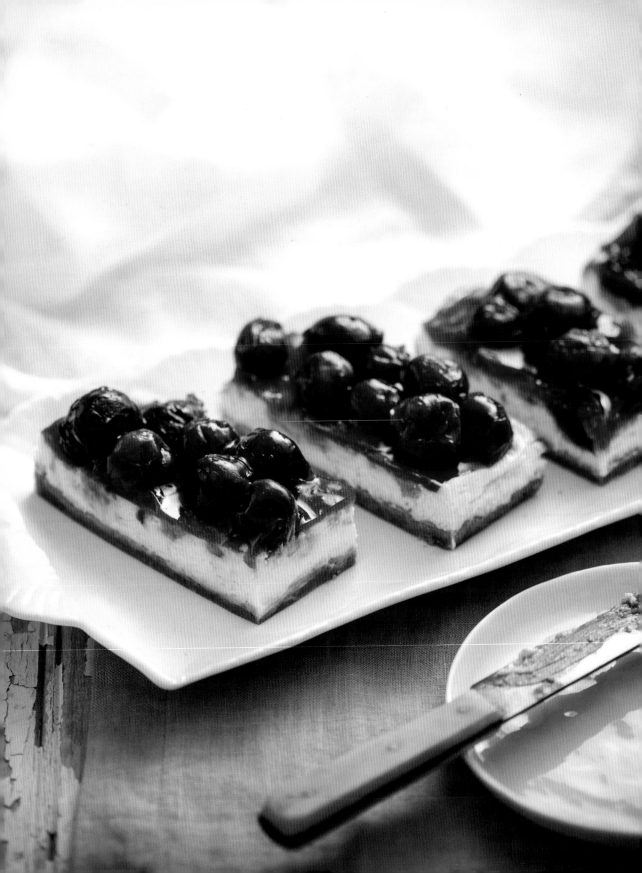

CHERRY CHEESECAKE BARS
WITH EXTRA GRAHAM CRUNCH

Cheesecake is always made with a graham-crumb crust, so why not use whole grain grahams and make the graham crust bigger and thicker, giving this creamy bar even more crunchy graham goodness? It's a dessert, to be sure, but it's lower in fat and higher in whole grains than many other sweets, so it's just a nudge toward the virtuous side of the scale.

SERVES 9 (MAKES 9 BARS)

3 sheets of whole grain graham crackers (27 sheets of crackers)

1/2 cup (1 stick) unsalted butter, melted, plus more for the pan

1/2 cup honey

1 (8-ounce) package Neufchâtel cheese, at room temperature

1 1/2 cups vanilla Greek yogurt (low-fat or nonfat is fine)

2 large eggs

1/2 cup granulated sugar

1 tablespoon freshly squeezed lemon juice

1 teaspoon vanilla extract

TOPPING

16 ounces frozen sweet cherries, thawed

1/4 cup granulated sugar

3/4 cup apple juice

2 tablespoons arrowroot

Preheat the oven to 350°F. Butter a 9-inch square pan.

In a food processor, pulse the grahams to a coarse crumb, then add the butter and honey and pulse to mix. Transfer one third of the mixture to a bowl and reserve for topping. Press the remaining two thirds of the crumbs into the prepared pan. Rinse and dry the food processor bowl, then add the Neufchâtel cheese and process until smooth, scraping once and repeating. Add the yogurt, eggs, sugar, lemon juice, and vanilla and process, scraping down and repeating until smooth and well mixed.

Pour the Neufchâtel mixture over the crust in the pan, then smooth the top. Sprinkle the reserved graham crumbs over the Neufchâtel layer and bake for 30 minutes, or until the cheese filling is puffed and jiggles only slightly when shaken.

In a saucepan, stir together the cherries, sugar, apple juice, and arrowroot until the arrowroot is dissolved. Bring to a boil and boil until thickened. Take off the heat and let cool slightly. Dollop over the pan of bars and spread to cover. Chill until set.

Slice 3 x 3 to make 9 bars. Keeps for 4 days in an airtight container in the refrigerator.

FUDGY BROWNIE CUPCAKES

For a full-on, gooey brownie experience, under-bake these just a little, then chill them. Buttery and chocolate rich, these cupcakes will answer your sweet tooth with a deep and dark satisfaction. Who cares about the whole grains?

SERVES 9

6 tablespoons unsalted butter

2 ounces semisweet chocolate, chopped

3 ounces unsweetened chocolate, chopped

1 cup packed light brown sugar

$1/8$ teaspoon salt

2 large eggs

1 teaspoon vanilla extract

$1/2$ cup whole wheat pastry flour

$1/4$ cup rye or buckwheat flour

Confectioners' sugar, for dusting

Preheat the oven to 350°F. Line 9 muffin cups of a muffin pan with paper liners.

In a double boiler or a metal bowl set over barely simmering water, combine the butter and chocolates. Stir occasionally, until melted and smooth. Take off the heat and cool to room temperature.

Stir the brown sugar, salt, eggs, and vanilla into the chocolate mixture. Mix well, then stir in the flours. Use a $1/4$-cup measure to scoop batter into the prepared muffin cups and divide any leftover batter between the cups.

Bake for 15 to 18 minutes, or until the cupcakes are puffed but still liquid in the center. Let cool in the pan for 10 minutes, then transfer cupcakes to a rack to cool. Serve at room temperature and store in the refrigerator for a fudgy texture. To serve, use a small wire strainer to sift confectioners' sugar over the cupcakes.

Keeps for 1 week, tightly covered, in the refrigerator.

ACKNOWLEDGMENTS

THIS COOKBOOK IS A LABOR OF LOVE AND I AM PROFOUNDLY GRATEFUL FOR ALL THE people who have helped make it the best that it can be. My number one food tester and husband, Stan, is my loyal cheerleader, and I could not do it without him. I'd like to give a collective big hug to all my recipe testers, including Lisa Genis, Kristine Vick, Lisa Scribner, and Melodie Bahan. For expert baking guidance and emotional support, I am grateful for Jill O'Connor, pastry chef supreme. For last-minute bread tips, Zoe Francois.

At Running Press, I am forever grateful for the skilled editing and support of Zachary Leibman and Kristen Green Wiewora. Thanks to photographer Steven Legato for making my words into an actual, beautiful book and Carrie Purcell and Mariellen Melker for food and prop styling. Also, thanks to Amanda Richmond for the wonderful design.

The inception and inspiration for this book was aided by my collaborations with Grains For Health Foundation, especially Dr. Len Marquardt, Beth Maschoff, and Denise Hauge. As always, the Whole Grains Council is a beacon of resources and education.

INDEX

Note: Page references in *italics* indicate recipe photographs.

A

Almond(s)
- -Apricot Spread, 158
- -Cherry Grain Pudding, 181
- -Cherry Quick Bread, 74, *75*
- Lemon-Strawberry Quinoa Breakfast Salad, *36*, 37
- –Sweet Cherry Granola, Super-Chunky, 32
- Whole Wheat Penne in Roasted-Pepper Romesco Sauce, 116

Amaranth
- about, 23
- cooking, 20

Antioxidants, 11

Apple Butter
- –Cinnamon Bars, 50
- –Swirl Cupcakes with Cider Glaze, 179

Apple(s)
- and Cheddar Graham Sams, 158
- Cinnamon–Apple Butter Bars, 50
- Pancake, Puffy Baked, 56
- Sautéed, Grilled Steel-Cut Oat Slabs with, 41
- Spinach Quattro Salad–Four Salads on One Plate, 84

Apricot(s)
- -Almond Spread, 158
- Date and Grain Energy Bars, 34
- Fruity Carrot Muffins, 51
- Oatmeal and Mixed-Fruit Jumbo Cookies, 175

Arsenic, concerns about, 21–22

Arugula-Ricotta Pesto, Whole Wheat Angel Hair with, 115

Asparagus
- Italian Farro and White Bean Salad with, *88*, 89
- Spring Veggie Stew with Bulgur, *102*, 103

Avocado(s)
- Blue Cheese, and Creamy Tomato Dressing, Mixed Rice Cobb with, 82
- Brown Rice California Rolls with Salmon, 151
- Buddha Bowls for Two, 81
- and Chipotle Grain and Turkey Wraps, 146
- and Mango, Lime Quinoa Salad with, 92, *93*
- Salsa, 133
- Sushi Broccoli and Brown Rice Salad, 90

B

Bacon, Smoky, and Grain Frittata, 148, *149*

Baking Mix, Make Your Own, 61

Baking-Mix Biscuits, 62

Baking-Mix Pancakes, 62

Baking-Mix Scones, 63

Banana(s)
- Blueberry Green Smoothie with Leftover Grain, 35
- -Strawberry Quinoa Smoothie, 35

Barley
- pearled, about, 23
- pearled, cooking, 20
- and Pecan Burgers with Peach Ketchup, *134*, 135
- and Sweet Potato Timbales, 128, *129*
- whole, about, 23
- whole, cooking, 20

Bars
- Cherry Cheesecake, with Extra Graham Crunch, *186*, 187
- Cinnamon–Apple Butter, 50
- Energy, Date and Grain, 34
- Light Buckwheat Brownies, *177*, 178

Basil
- Baked Polenta Rounds, Easy, 114
- Italian Bread Salad, 80
- Pesto Turkey Loaf with Oats, 142
- Spinach Quattro Salad–Four Salads on One Plate, 84

Bean(s)
- Black, Burgers, Easy, with Oats and Avocado Salsa, 133
- Black, Quesadillas, Easy, with Raspberry-Kiwi Salsa, 143

Cornbread-Topped Chili Casserole, 152–53
Easy Edamame Hummus, 162
Quick Veggie Chili with Mushrooms
    and Bulgur, 97
Savory Porridge, 45
White, and Farro Salad with Asparagus,
    Italian, *88*, 89
Beet(s)
    and Buckwheat Borscht with Parsley-Yogurt
        Garnish, 104, *105*
    Buddha Bowls for Two, 81
Berry(ies). *See also specific berries*
    Big Cinnamon-Oat Pancakes with, 57
    -Nectarine Crumble, Quick Stovetop, 174
    Pomegranate, and Nuts, Overnight Oat
        Soak with, *28*, 29
Biryani, Indian Yellow Mixed-Grain, *124*, 125
Biscuits, Baking-Mix, 62
Biscuit-Topped Breakfast Pie, 55
Blueberry Green Smoothie with Leftover Grain, 35
Breadcrumbs, Garlicky, Kale, and Parmesan,
    Whole Wheat Spaghetti with, 117
Breads
    Fruity Carrot Muffins, 51
    Yogurt–Cottage Cheese Muffins with
        Tarragon, 52
Bread(s). *See also* Croutons
    Baking-Mix Biscuits, 62
    Baking-Mix Scones, 63
    buying, 14
    Cheddar-Chive Cornbread, *72*, 73
    Cherry and Pine Nut Breakfast Focaccia, 53
    Cinnamon Toast and Fruit "Caprese," 46
    Cinnamon Toasts with Yogurt Dip, 161
    No-Knead "Stealth," 64, *65*
    Parsley-Parmesan Popovers, *76*, 77
    Pudding, Savory Spinach and Cheese, 120
    Quick, Cherry-Almond, 74, *75*
    Quick, Savory Spinach, 71
    Salad, Italian, 80
    Soft Buttermilk Buns, 68
    Stuffing, Herbed, 113
    whole wheat, tips for, 66

Broccoli
    and Brown Rice Salad, Sushi, 90
    Smoky Bacon and Grain Frittata, 148, *149*
    Whole Wheat Angel Hair with Arugula-Ricotta
        Pesto, 115
Brownie Cupcakes, Fudgy, 188
Brownies, Light Buckwheat, *177*, 178
Buckwheat (flour)
    about, 24
    Brownies, Light, *177*, 178
Buckwheat (groats)
    about, 24
    and Beet Borscht with Parsley-Yogurt
        Garnish, 104, *105*
    cooking, 20
    "Raw" Cookie Dough Bites, 173
    Savory Granola Croutons for Salad or Soup, 69
    Savory Kasha with Parsnips, 122, *123*
Bulgur
    about, 24
    cooking, 20
    Herbed Bread Stuffing, 113
    Herb Pilaf, Easy, 111
    and Mushrooms, Quick Veggie Chili with, 97
    Spring Veggie Stew with, *102*, 103
Burgers
    Easy Black Bean, with Oats and
        Avocado Salsa, 133
    Pecan and Barley, with Peach Ketchup, *134*, 135
Buttermilk
    Buns, Soft, 68
    Creamy, Party Mix, 160
    Dressing, Wheat Berry and Shredded
        Cabbage Salad with, 85

C

Cabbage
    Shredded, and Wheat Berry Salad with
        Buttermilk Dressing, 85
    Soup, Spicy, with Leftover-Grain Dumplings, 109
    Veggie and Brown Rice Medley, 126
Cakes
    Apple Butter–Swirl Cupcakes with
        Cider Glaze, 179
    Coffee, Peachy Yogurt, 48, *49*
    Cranberry Cornmeal Upside-Down, *182*, 183

Cakes (*continued*)
    Fudgy Brownie Cupcakes, 188
    Orange-Raspberry Bundt, 184, *185*
    Peanut Butter, with Chocolate Frosting, 180
Carrot(s)
    Biscuit-Topped Breakfast Pie, 55
    Brown Rice California Rolls with Salmon, 151
    Egg Curry Breakfast Bowl, *42,* 43
    Lemon-Strawberry Quinoa Breakfast Salad, *36,* 37
    -Millet Soup, Creamy Curried, with Mint, 98, *99*
    Muffins, Fruity, 51
    Roasted, Cauliflower, and Parmesan Croutons
      over Spinach, 83
    Soba or Whole Wheat Spaghetti with Sesame
      Dressing and Sugar Snap Peas, 91
    Wheat Berry and Shredded Cabbage Salad with
      Buttermilk Dressing, 85
Cauliflower
    Indian Yellow Mixed-Grain Biryani, *124,* 125
    Roasted, Carrots, and Parmesan Croutons
      over Spinach, 83
    Spinach Quiche, Grain-Crust, 147
Cereals
    Boil-and-Leave Steel-Cut Oats, 30
    buying, 14
    Daily Walnut-Raisin Olive Oil Granola, 33
    making ahead, 17–18
    Overnight Oat Soak with Pomegranate, Berries,
      and Nuts, *28,* 29
    Quick Stovetop Granola, 31
    Savory Porridge, 45
    Super-Chunky Sweet Cherry–Almond
      Granola, 32
Cheese
    Apples and Cheddar Graham Sams, 158
    Barley and Sweet Potato Timbales, 128, *129*
    Basic Croutons with Variations, 70
    Blue, Avocados, and Creamy Tomato Dressing,
    Mixed Rice Cobb with, 82
    Breakfast Pizza with Strawberry Sauce, Ricotta,
      and Sweet Walnut "Meatballs," 54
    Cheddar-Chive Cornbread, *72,* 73
    Cherry Cheesecake Bars with Extra Graham
      Crunch, *186,* 187
    Cinnamon Toast and Fruit "Caprese," 46
    Cottage, –Yogurt Muffins with Tarragon, 52
    Easy Basil Baked Polenta Rounds, 114

Grain-Crust Spinach Cauliflower Quiche, 147
    Kale and Tomato Caesar Salad, *78,* 79
    Maple Ricotta with Mini Chocolate Chips, 158
    Parmesan Corn, 157
    Parsley-Parmesan Popovers, *76,* 77
    Quinoa and Sun-Dried Tomato Timbales, 130
    Quinoa-Feta Phyllo Triangles, 136
    Rice Cake Tuna Melts, 168
    Roasted Cauliflower, Carrots, and Parmesan
      Croutons over Spinach, 83
    Savory Oatmeal Cookies with Cheddar, 169
    Smoky Bacon and Grain Frittata, 148, *149*
    and Spinach Bread Pudding, Savory, 120
    Spinach Quattro Salad–Four Salads on
      One Plate, 84
    Whole Grain Mac and, with Peas, *118,* 119
    Whole Wheat Angel Hair with Arugula-
      Ricotta Pesto, 115
    Whole Wheat Pita Pizzas, 164, *165*
    Whole Wheat Spaghetti with Garlicky
      Breadcrumbs, Kale, and Parmesan, 117
Cherry(ies)
    -Almond Grain Pudding, 181
    -Almond Quick Bread, 74, *75*
    Cheesecake Bars with Extra Graham
      Crunch, *186,* 187
    Oatmeal and Mixed-Fruit Jumbo Cookies, 175
    and Pine Nut Breakfast Focaccia, 53
    Sweet, –Almond Granola, Super-Chunky, 32
Chex, Whole Grain Cracker, and Nut Mixes, 160
Chicken
    Biscuit-Topped Breakfast Pie, 55
    Fingers, Crunchy-Crumb, with Honey
      Mustard, 150
    Soup, Fast, with Quinoa, 101
Chili, Quick Veggie, with Mushrooms and Bulgur, 97
Chili Casserole, Cornbread-Topped, 152–53
Chocolate
    Baking-Mix Scones, 63
    Chips, Mini, Maple Ricotta with, 158
    Cookies, Chewy, 176, *177*
    Frosting, 180
    Fudgy Brownie Cupcakes, 188
    Graham Cracker and Pudding "Pie," 159
    Granola Bark, 171
    Hazelnut Spread, 158
    Light Buckwheat Brownies, *177,* 178

"Raw" Cookie Dough Bites, 173
Chowder, Millet-Corn, with Chipotle, 107
Cinnamon
    –Apple Butter Bars, 50
    Corn, *156,* 157
    -Oat Pancakes, Big, with Berries, 57
    Toast and Fruit "Caprese," 46
    Toasts with Yogurt Dip, 161
Clementines and Yogurt Dressing, Farro with, 38, *39*
Coffee Cake, Peachy Yogurt, 48, *49*
Colon cancer, 11
Cookie Dough Bites, "Raw," 173
Cookies. *See also* Bars
    Chocolate, Chewy, 176, *177*
    Oatmeal and Mixed-Fruit Jumbo, 175
    Savory Oatmeal, with Cheddar, 169
Corn
    -Millet Chowder with Chipotle, 107
    Spinach Quattro Salad–Four Salads on
      One Plate, 84
Corn Chips, Baked, with Easy Edamame
  Hummus, 162
Cornmeal
    Cheddar-Chive Cornbread, *72,* 73
    Cornbread-Topped Chili Casserole, 152–53
    Cranberry Upside-Down Cake, *182,* 183
    Crunchy-Crumb Chicken Fingers with Honey
      Mustard, 150
    Easy Basil Baked Polenta Rounds, 114
Couscous
    about, 24
    cooking, 20
    Quick Lemony, with Spinach, 112
Cracker, Whole Grain, Chex, and Nut Mixes, 160
Crackers, buying, 14
Cranberry(ies)
    Cornmeal Upside-Down Cake, *182,* 183
    Savory Oatmeal Cookies with Cheddar, 169
Croquettes, Potato-Grain, with Warm
  Honey-Mustard Sauce, 131
Croutons
    Basic, with Variations, 70
    Parmesan, Roasted Cauliflower, and
      Carrots over Spinach, 83
Cucumber(s)
    Brown Rice California Rolls with Salmon, 151
    Italian Bread Salad, 80

-Lime Salsa, 138, *139*
    Middle Eastern Freekeh Salad with Sesame-
      Yogurt Dressing, 86, *87*
    Soba or Whole Wheat Spaghetti with Sesame
      Dressing and Sugar Snap Peas, 91
Cupcakes
    Apple Butter–Swirl, with Cider Glaze, 179
    Fudgy Brownie, 188
Curried Carrot-Millet Soup, Creamy,
  with Mint, 98, *99*
Curry, Egg, Breakfast Bowl, *42,* 43
Curry Ketchup, Leftover-Grain Scallion
  Cakes with, 166, *167*

D

Date and Grain Energy Bars, 34
Diabetes, 10
Dips and spreads
    Almond-Apricot Spread, 158
    Chocolate Hazelnut, 158
    Easy Edamame Hummus, 162
    Maple Ricotta with Mini Chocolate Chips, 158
    Yogurt Dip, 161
Dumplings, Leftover-Grain, Spicy Cabbage
  Soup with, 109

E

Egg(s)
    Curry Breakfast Bowl, *42,* 43
    Japanese Breakfast Bowl, 43
    Leftover-Grain Omelets and Scrambles, 40
    Savory Porridge, 45
    Smoky Bacon and Grain Frittata, 148, *149*
    and Veggies, Any-Grain Fried "Rice" with, 127

F

Farro
    with Clementines and Yogurt Dressing, 38, *39*
    cooking, 20
    and White Bean Salad with Asparagus, Italian,
      88, 89
Fish
    Baked Sole Filled with Lemony Dill Pilaf, 140
    Brown Rice California Rolls with Salmon, 151
    Cakes, Lime, with Brown Rice and Dipping
      Sauce, 137

Fish (*continued*)
    Japanese Breakfast Bowl, 43
    Red Quinoa–Crusted Baked, with Cucumber-
        Lime Salsa, 138, *139*
    Rice Cake Tuna Melts, 168
    Savory Porridge, 45
Flours. *See also* Whole wheat flour
    glossary of, 23–27
    swapping, note about, 66
Focaccia, Cherry and Pine Nut Breakfast, 53
Fonio, about, 24
Freekeh
    about, 25
    cooking, 20
    Salad, Middle Eastern, with Sesame-Yogurt
        Dressing, 86, *87*
Frittata, Smoky Bacon and Grain, 148, *149*
Frosting, Chocolate, 180
Fruit. *See also specific fruits*
    Baking-Mix Scones, 63
    Seasonal, Yogurt-Granola Parfait with, 163
    Yogurt Dip, 161

G

Glycemic impact, 11
Graham Cracker(s)
    buying, 14
    Cherry Cheesecake Bars with Extra Graham
        Crunch, *186,* 187
    Graham Sams, 158
    and Pudding "Pie," 159
Grain(s). *See also specific grains*
    Any-, Fried "Rice" with Veggies and Egg, 127
    buying in bulk, 17
    buying 100% whole grain products, 14–15
    cooked, freezing, 17
    cooking, in pressure cooker, 22–23
    cooking, in rice cooker, 22
    cooking, in slow cooker, 22
    cooking, pasta-style, 18
    cooking ahead, 17
    cooking chart, 20
    cooking methods, 19
    cooking porridge-style, 44
    cooking risotto-style, 44
    dry-toasting, 29
    fast-cooking, 15–16
    freezing whole grain foods, 18
    glossary of, 23–27
    health benefits, 7–9, 10–11
    incorporating into meals, 12–13
    Leftover-, Omelets and Scrambles, 40
    Leftover-, Scallion Cakes with Curry
        Ketchup, 166, *167*
    longer-cooking, 16
    sautéing, 29
    soaking, 21
    swapping, in recipes, 18–19
    USDA recommendations, 7
Granola
    Bark, 171
    Brittle Chunks, 172
    Croutons, Savory, for Salad or Soup, 69
    Island Smoothie, 35
    Quick Stovetop, 31
    Super-Chunky Sweet Cherry–Almond, 32
    Walnut-Raisin Olive Oil, Daily, 33
    -Yogurt Parfait with Seasonal Fruit, 163
Greens. *See also* Kale; Spinach
    Beet and Buckwheat Borscht with Parsley-
        Yogurt Garnish, 104, *105*
    Fast Chicken Soup with Quinoa, 101
    Japanese Breakfast Bowl, 43
    Mixed Rice Cobb with Avocados, Blue Cheese,
        and Creamy Tomato Dressing, 82
    Whole Wheat Angel Hair with Arugula-
        Ricotta Pesto, 115

H

Hazelnut Chocolate Spread, 158
Healthy food, psychology of, 12–13
Heart disease, 10
Honey
    Mustard, Crunchy-Crumb Chicken
        Fingers with, 150
    -Mustard Sauce, Warm, Potato-Grain
        Croquettes with, 131
Hummus, Easy Edamame, 162

I

Inflammation, 10
Intestinal wall permeability ("leaky gut"), 10

K

Kale
    Buddha Bowls for Two, 81
    Fast Chicken Soup with Quinoa, 101
    Garlicky Breadcrumbs, and Parmesan,
        Whole Wheat Spaghetti with, 117
    Smoky Bacon and Grain Frittata, 148, *149*
    and Tomato Caesar Salad, *78, 79*
Kamut, cooking, 20
Kañiwa
    about, 25
    cooking, 20
Kasha with Parsnips, Savory, 122, *123*
Ketchup
    Curry, Leftover-Grain Scallion Cakes
        with, 166, *167*
    Peach, 135
Kiwi-Raspberry Salsa, 143

L

Labels, reading, 15
Lemony Couscous, Quick, with Spinach, 112
Lemony Dill Pilaf, Baked Sole Filled with, 140
Lime
    -Cucumber Salsa, 138, *139*
    Fish Cakes with Brown Rice and Dipping
        Sauce, 137
    Quinoa Salad with Avocado and Mango, 92, *93*
    Thai Chili Party Mix, 160

M

Mango and Avocado, Lime Quinoa Salad with, 92, *93*
Maple (syrup)
    Graham Cracker and Pudding "Pie," 159
    -Pear Sauce, Overnight Whole Wheat Waffles
        with, *58,* 59
    Ricotta with Mini Chocolate Chips, 158
Meat. *See* Pork
"Meatballs"
    Grain and Nut Balls with Marinara and
        Whole Wheat Penne, 141
    Sweet Walnut, Strawberry Sauce, and Ricotta,
        Breakfast Pizza with, 54
Millet
    about, 25

Blueberry Green Smoothie with
    Leftover Grain, 35
Breakfast Pizza with Strawberry Sauce, Ricotta,
    and Sweet Walnut "Meatballs," 54
-Carrot Soup, Creamy Curried, with Mint, 98, *99*
cooking, 20
-Corn Chowder with Chipotle, 107
Date and Grain Energy Bars, 34
Spicy Cabbage Soup with Leftover-Grain
    Dumplings, 109
Mint
    Creamy Curried Carrot-Millet Soup with, 98, *99*
    Indian Yellow Mixed-Grain Biryani, *124,* 125
    Middle Eastern Freekeh Salad with Sesame-
        Yogurt Dressing, 86, *87*
Muffins
    Fruity Carrot, 51
    Yogurt–Cottage Cheese, with Tarragon, 52
Mushrooms
    and Bulgur, Quick Veggie Chili with, 97
    Cornbread-Topped Chili Casserole, 152–53
    Savory Spinach and Cheese Bread Pudding, 120
Mustard
    Honey, Crunchy-Crumb Chicken Fingers
        with, 150
    -Honey Sauce, Warm, Potato-Grain
        Croquettes with, 131

N

Nectarine-Berry Crumble, Quick Stovetop, 174
Nut(s). *See also* Almond(s); Peanuts; Walnut(s)
    Baking-Mix Scones, 63
    Chocolate Hazelnut Spread, 158
    Pecan and Barley Burgers with Peach Ketchup,
        134, 135
    Pine, and Cherry Breakfast Focaccia, 53
    Pomegranate, and Berries, Overnight Oat
        Soak with, *28, 29*
    Whole Grain Cracker, and Chex Mixes, 160

O

Oat groats, cooking, 20
Oat(s)
    about, 25
    Breakfast Pizza with Strawberry Sauce,
        Ricotta, and Sweet Walnut "Meatballs," 54

Oat(s) (*continued*)
    Chewy Chocolate Cookies, 176, *177*
    Cinnamon–Apple Butter Bars, 50
    -Cinnamon Pancakes, Big, with Berries, 57
    cooking, 20
    Cornbread-Topped Chili Casserole, 152–53
    Crust, Savory Streusel Squash Pie with, *144,* 145
    Daily Walnut-Raisin Olive Oil Granola, 33
    Date and Grain Energy Bars, 34
    Easy Black Bean Burgers with, and Avocado
      Salsa, 133
    Granola Brittle Chunks, 172
    Oatmeal and Mixed-Fruit Jumbo Cookies, 175
    Pesto Turkey Loaf with, 142
    Quick Stovetop Granola, 31
    Quick Stovetop Nectarine-Berry Crumble, 174
    Savory Granola Croutons for Salad or Soup, 69
    Savory Oatmeal Cookies with Cheddar, 169
    Soak, Overnight, with Pomegranate, Berries,
      and Nuts, *28, 29*
    Soft Buttermilk Buns, 68
    Steel-Cut, Boil-and-Leave, 30
    Steel-Cut, Pumpkin Pie Baked, 47
    Steel-Cut, Slabs, Grilled, with Sautéed Apples, 41
    Super-Chunky Sweet Cherry–Almond Granola, 32
Omelets and Scrambles, Leftover-Grain, 40
Orange-Raspberry Bundt, 184, *185*

P

Pancakes
    Baking-Mix, 62
    Big Cinnamon-Oat, with Berries, 57
    Puffy Baked Apple, 56
Parfait, Yogurt-Granola, with Seasonal Fruit, 163
Parsley
    Italian Bread Salad, 80
    Middle Eastern Freekeh Salad with Sesame-
      Yogurt Dressing, 86, *87*
    -Parmesan Popovers, *76,* 77
    -Yogurt Garnish, Beet and Buckwheat Borscht
      with, 104, *105*
Parsnips, Savory Kasha with, 122, *123*
Party Mixes, 160
Pasta and noodles
    Grain and Nut Balls with Marinara and Whole
      Wheat Penne, 141

    Soba or Whole Wheat Spaghetti with Sesame
      Dressing and Sugar Snap Peas, 91
    whole grain, buying, 14
    Whole Grain Mac and Cheese with Peas, *118,* 119
    Whole Grain Sour Cream with Dill Noodles, 121
    Whole Wheat Angel Hair with Arugula-Ricotta
      Pesto, 115
    Whole Wheat Penne in Roasted-Pepper Romesco
      Sauce, 116
    Whole Wheat Spaghetti with Garlicky
      Breadcrumbs, Kale, and Parmesan, 117
Peach(es)
    Ketchup, 135
    Peachy Yogurt Coffee Cake, 48, *49*
Peanut Butter
    Cake with Chocolate Frosting, 180
    Corn, 155
Peanuts
    Creamy Buttermilk Party Mix, 160
    Indian Yellow Mixed-Grain Biryani, *124,* 125
    Thai Chili Lime Party Mix, 160
Pear(s)
    Cinnamon Toast and Fruit "Caprese," 46
    -Maple Sauce, Overnight Whole Wheat Waffles
      with, *58,* 59
    Wild Rice, and Roasted Sweet Potato Salad
      with Walnuts, *94,* 95
Peas
    Any-Grain Fried "Rice" with Veggies and Egg, 127
    Indian Yellow Mixed-Grain Biryani, *124,* 125
    Sugar Snap, and Sesame Dressing, Soba or Whole
      Wheat Spaghetti with, 91
    Whole Grain Mac and Cheese with, *118,* 119
Pecan and Barley Burgers with Peach
  Ketchup, *134,* 135
Pepper(s)
    Avocado Salsa, 133
    Chipotle and Avocado Grain and Turkey
      Wraps, 146
    Mexican Tortilla Soup with Shrimp, 108
    Quick Veggie Chili with Mushrooms and
      Bulgur, 97
    Roasted- , Romesco Sauce, Whole Wheat
      Penne in, 116
Pesto
    Arugula-Ricotta, Whole Wheat Angel Hair
      with, 115

Turkey Loaf with Oats, 142
Phyllo Triangles, Quinoa-Feta, 136
"Pie," Graham Cracker and Pudding, 159
Pies
    Breakfast, Biscuit-Topped, 55
    Squash, Savory Streusel, with Oat Crust, *144,* 145
Pilaf, Easy Bulgur Herb, 111
Pine Nut and Cherry Breakfast Focaccia, 53
Pizza Dough, Overnight "Stealth," 67
Pizzas
    Breakfast, with Strawberry Sauce, Ricotta,
      and Sweet Walnut "Meatballs," 54
    Whole Wheat Pita, 164, *165*
Polenta Rounds, Easy Basil Baked, 114
Pomegranate, Berries, and Nuts, Overnight
  Oat Soak with, *28, 29*
Popcorns, Super, 155–57, *156*
Popovers, Parsley-Parmesan, *76,* 77
Pork
    Smoky Bacon and Grain Frittata, 148, *149*
    Spicy Cabbage Soup with Leftover-Grain
      Dumplings, 109
Porridge, Savory, 45
Potatoes, sweet. *See* Sweet Potato(es)
Potato-Grain Croquettes with Warm
  Honey-Mustard Sauce, 131
Poultry. *See* Chicken; Turkey
Prebiotics, 11
Pressure cookers, 22–23
Pretzels, buying, 14
Pudding
    Cherry-Almond Grain, 181
    and Graham Cracker "Pie," 159
Pumpkin Pie Baked Steel-Cut Oats, 47

Q

Quesadillas, Easy Black Bean, with
  Raspberry-Kiwi Salsa, 143
Quiche, Grain-Crust Spinach Cauliflower, 147
Quinoa
    about, 26
    Chipotle and Avocado Grain and
      Turkey Wraps, 146
    cooking, 20
    Fast Chicken Soup with, 101
    -Feta Phyllo Triangles, 136

Japanese Breakfast Bowl, 43
Lemon-Strawberry Breakfast Salad, *36,* 37
Lime Salad with Avocado and Mango, 92, *93*
Red, –Crusted Baked Fish with Cucumber-Lime
  Salsa, 138, *139*
Smoothie, Strawberry-Banana, 35
and Sun-Dried Tomato Timbales, 130

R

Raisin(s)
    Indian Yellow Mixed-Grain Biryani, *124,* 125
    Oatmeal and Mixed-Fruit Jumbo Cookies, 175
    -Walnut Olive Oil Granola, Daily, 33
Raspberry(ies)
    Cinnamon Toast and Fruit "Caprese," 46
    -Kiwi Salsa, 143
    -Orange Bundt, 184, *185*
Rice
    Baked Sole Filled with Lemony Dill Pilaf, 140
    black, cooking, 20
    brown, about, 26
    brown, and arsenic, 21–22
    Brown, and Broccoli Salad, Sushi, 90
    Brown, and Veggie Medley, 126
    Brown, California Rolls with Salmon, 151
    brown, cooking, 20
    Brown, Lime Fish Cakes with, and Dipping
      Sauce, 137
    Buddha Bowls for Two, 81
    Cherry-Almond Grain Pudding, 181
    Creamy Spinach Soup, 100
    Egg Curry Breakfast Bowl, *42,* 43
    Grain and Nut Balls with Marinara and
      Whole Wheat Penne, 141
    Grain-Crust Spinach Cauliflower Quiche, 147
    Indian Yellow Mixed-Grain Biryani, *124,* 125
    Mixed, Cobb with Avocados, Blue Cheese,
      and Creamy Tomato Dressing, 82
    Potato-Grain Croquettes with Warm Honey-
      Mustard Sauce, 131
    red, cooking, 20
    Savory Porridge, 45
    whole grain, about, 26
    Wild, Pear, and Roasted Sweet Potato Salad
      with Walnuts, *94,* 95
Rice Cake Tuna Melts, 168

Rice cookers, electric, 22
"Rice" Fried, Any-Grain, with Veggies and Egg, 127
Rye
    about, 26
    berries, cooking, 20

S

Salads
    Bread, Italian, 80
    Breakfast, Lemon-Strawberry Quinoa, *36, 37*
    Buddha Bowls for Two, 81
    Farro with Clementines and Yogurt
        Dressing, 38, *39*
    Freekeh, Middle Eastern, with Sesame-Yogurt
        Dressing, 86, *87*
    Italian Farro and White Bean, with Asparagus,
        88, 89
    Kale and Tomato Caesar, *78,* 79
    Lime Quinoa, with Avocado and Mango, 92, *93*
    Mixed Rice Cobb with Avocados, Blue Cheese,
        and Creamy Tomato Dressing, 82
    Roasted Cauliflower, Carrots, and Parmesan
        Croutons over Spinach, 83
    Savory Granola Croutons for, 69
    Spinach Quattro, –Four Salads on One Plate, 84
    Sushi Broccoli and Brown Rice, 90
    Wheat Berry and Shredded Cabbage, with
        Buttermilk Dressing, 85
    Wild Rice, Pear, and Roasted Sweet Potato,
        with Walnuts, *94,* 95
Salmon
    Brown Rice California Rolls with, 151
    Japanese Breakfast Bowl, 43
    Lime Fish Cakes with Brown Rice and
        Dipping Sauce, 137
Salsas
    Avocado, 133
    Cucumber-Lime, 138, *139*
    Raspberry-Kiwi, 143
Sausages
    Biscuit-Topped Breakfast Pie, 55
    Spicy Cabbage Soup with Leftover-Grain
        Dumplings, 109
Scallion Leftover-Grain Cakes with
    Curry Ketchup, 166, *167*
Scones, Baking-Mix, 63

Seafood. *See* Fish; Shrimp
Sesame seeds
    Lime Fish Cakes with Brown Rice and
        Dipping Sauce, 137
    Savory Granola Croutons for Salad or Soup, 69
Shrimp, Mexican Tortilla Soup with, 108
Slow cookers, 22
Smoothies
    Blueberry Green, with Leftover Grain, 35
    Granola Island, 35
    Strawberry-Banana Quinoa, 35
Snacks, whole grain, buying, 14
Sole, Baked, Filled with Lemony Dill Pilaf, 140
Soups
    Beet and Buckwheat Borscht with Parsley-
        Yogurt Garnish, 104, *105*
    Cabbage, Spicy, with Leftover-Grain
        Dumplings, 109
    Chicken, Fast, with Quinoa, 101
    Curried Carrot-Millet, Creamy, with Mint, 98, *99*
    Millet-Corn Chowder with Chipotle, 107
    Quick Veggie Chili with Mushrooms and
        Bulgur, 97
    Savory Granola Croutons for, 69
    Spinach, Creamy, 100
    Spring Veggie Stew with Bulgur, *102,* 103
    Tomato-Zucchini, Summer, with Wheat
        Berries, 106
    Tortilla, Mexican, with Shrimp, 108
Spinach
    Barley and Sweet Potato Timbales, 128, *129*
    Biscuit-Topped Breakfast Pie, 55
    Blueberry Green Smoothie with Leftover
        Grain, 35
    Cauliflower Quiche, Grain-Crust, 147
    and Cheese Bread Pudding, Savory, 120
    Fast Chicken Soup with Quinoa, 101
    Granola Island Smoothie, 35
    Japanese Breakfast Bowl, 43
    Quattro Salad–Four Salads on One Plate, 84
    Quick Bread, Savory, 71
    Quick Lemony Couscous with, 112
    Quinoa-Feta Phyllo Triangles, 136
    Roasted Cauliflower, Carrots, and Parmesan
        Croutons over, 83
    Soup, Creamy, 100
    Whole Wheat Pita Pizzas, 164, *165*

Squash. *See also* Zucchini
    Pie, Savory Streusel, with Oat Crust, *144,* 145
    Pumpkin Pie Baked Steel-Cut Oats, 47
Stealth nutrition, 12–13
Strawberry(ies)
    -Banana Quinoa Smoothie, 35
    Graham Cracker and Pudding "Pie," 159
    Granola Island Smoothie, 35
    -Lemon Quinoa Breakfast Salad, *36,* 37
    Sauce, Ricotta, and Sweet Walnut "Meatballs,"
      Breakfast Pizza with, 54
Strokes, 10
Stuffing, Herbed Bread, 113
Sunflower seeds
    Mixed Rice Cobb with Avocados, Blue Cheese,
      and Creamy Tomato Dressing, 82
    Savory Granola Croutons for Salad or Soup, 69
Sweet Potato(es)
    and Barley Timbales, 128, *129*
    Pecan and Barley Burgers with Peach
      Ketchup, *134,* 135
    Roasted, Wild Rice, and Pear Salad with
      Walnuts, *94,* 95
    Whole Grain Mac and Cheese with Peas, *118,* 119

T

Tahini
    Easy Edamame Hummus, 162
    Middle Eastern Freekeh Salad with Sesame-
      Yogurt Dressing, 86, *87*
    Soba or Whole Wheat Spaghetti with Sesame
      Dressing and Sugar Snap Peas, 91
Teff
    about, 27
    cooking, 20
Thai Chili Lime Party Mix, 160
Timbales
    Barley and Sweet Potato, 128, *129*
    Quinoa and Sun-Dried Tomato, 130
Tofu
    Buddha Bowls for Two, 81
    Graham Cracker and Pudding "Pie," 159
    Savory Porridge, 45
Tomato(es)
    Avocado Salsa, 133
    Chipotle and Avocado Grain and Turkey

Wraps, 146
    Dressing, Creamy, Avocados, and Blue Cheese,
      Mixed Rice Cobb with, 82
    Egg Curry Breakfast Bowl, *42, 43*
    Grain and Nut Balls with Marinara and
      Whole Wheat Penne, 141
    Italian Bread Salad, 80
    and Kale Caesar Salad, *78, 79*
    Rice Cake Tuna Melts, 168
    Spinach Quattro Salad–Four Salads on
      One Plate, 84
    Sun-Dried, and Quinoa Timbales, 130
    Whole Wheat Angel Hair with Arugula-
      Ricotta Pesto, 115
    Whole Wheat Pita Pizzas, 164, *165*
    -Zucchini Soup, Summer, with Wheat
      Berries, 106
Tortilla(s)
    Baked Corn Chips with Easy Edamame
      Hummus, 162
    Chipotle and Avocado Grain and Turkey
      Wraps, 146
    Easy Black Bean Quesadillas with Raspberry-
      Kiwi Salsa, 143
    Soup, Mexican, with Shrimp, 108
Tuna Melts, Rice Cake, 168
Turkey
    and Chipotle and Avocado Grain Wraps, 146
    Loaf, Pesto, with Oats, 142
    Savory Porridge, 45

V

Vegetables. *See also specific vegetables*
    Leftover-Grain Omelets and Scrambles, 40
    Savory Porridge, 45
    Spring Veggie Stew with Bulgur, *102,* 103
    Veggie and Brown Rice Medley, 126

W

Waffles, Overnight Whole Wheat, with
  Maple-Pear Sauce, *58,* 59
Walnut(s)
    Grain and Nut Balls with Marinara and
      Whole Wheat Penne, 141
    "Meatballs," Sweet, Strawberry Sauce, and
      Ricotta, Breakfast Pizza with, 54

Walnut(s) (*continued*)

    Quick Stovetop Granola, 31

    -Raisin Olive Oil Granola, Daily, 33

    Savory Granola Croutons for Salad or Soup, 69

    Savory Streusel Squash Pie with Oat Crust,
      144, 145

    Wild Rice, Pear, and Roasted Sweet Potato
      Salad with, *94,* 95

Weight maintenance, 10

Wheat Berry(ies)

    and Shredded Cabbage Salad with
      Buttermilk Dressing, 85

    Smoky Bacon and Grain Frittata, 148, *149*

    Spinach Quattro Salad–Four Salads on
      One Plate, 84

    Summer Tomato-Zucchini Soup with, 106

Whole wheat, cooking, 20

Whole wheat flour

    breads made with, note about, 66

    pastry, about, 13

    replacing white flour with, note about, 66

    white whole wheat, about, 13, 66

Wraps, Chipotle and Avocado Grain and Turkey, 146

Y

Yogurt

    Chocolate Frosting, 180

    Coffee Cake, Peachy, 48, *49*

    –Cottage Cheese Muffins with Tarragon, 52

    Dip, 161

    Dressing and Clementines, Farro with, 38, *39*

    -Granola Parfait with Seasonal Fruit, 163

    -Parsley Garnish, Beet and Buckwheat Borscht
      with, 104, *105*

    -Sesame Dressing, Middle Eastern Freekeh
      Salad with, 86, *87*

Z

Zucchini

    Mexican Tortilla Soup with Shrimp, 108

    -Tomato Soup, Summer, with Wheat Berries, 106